Healing Mind and Spirit: Introduction to Wild Card Therapy

Healing Mind and Spirit: Introduction to Wild Card Therapy

by Aunt T' Pathfinder & G. M. Blackman

BURMANBOOKS
.com

Published by BurmanBooks Inc.
4 Lamay Cres. Scarborough, Ontario Canada M1X 1J1

BB
BURMANBOOKS
.com

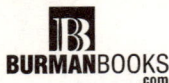

Pathfinder, Aunt T' & Blackman, G. M.
Healing Mind and Spirit: Introduction to Wild Card Therapy /
Aunt T' Pathfinder & G. M. Blackman

Cover Art by Aunt T' Pathfinder
Cover Design by www.AliveDesign.com

Edited by Solidus Communications www.solidus.ca

Typesetting by TypeWorx

Distribution:

North America: Independent Publishers Group,
814 North Franklin Street,
Chicago, Ill 60610

Printed in Canada

ISBN 0-9739097-0-6

The road for us both has been a truly fulfilling one
and one that many have contributed to.
Many thanks to family and friends who gave us patience,
including Jasmin and Simone for their creative input for the cover;
to Gisella Zukausky for helping Aunt at the beginning of her journey;
to our friends, Tracy M and Tracy C, without whom
we would still be wandering in the wilderness;
to mediumysticss.com staff and guests
who allowed us to refine our techniques on them;
to all at BurmanBooks for believing in us;
and to the True Creator and Angels for helping us always.

Table of Contents

Preface

The Wild Cards are spiritual tools and can be modified or refined to work best for each individual who has need of them, as long as they are being used to heal or cleanse. If they are used to attempt to cause harm to yourself or others, the energies and Beings beyond the material world (angels and such) who watch after and protect them, will rebound that wrongful energy, and regard your wrongful use of the Wild Cards as permission to cleanse you of that which has caused you to attempt wrongful use. Part of using the Wild Cards is also the cleansing commands you'll find in this book, and once you get to know them, all you need to do is call upon "all appropriate Wild Card Therapy commands to activate" to get the job done, without needing to go through them step by step. It's that simple.

Using the Wild Cards (depicted in future decks) is simple, but the creation of them is a story in itself. The truth is, they shaped me as much as I shaped them. In the beginning of their creation, I drew them as most artists draw, trying to capture what was in my mind's eye. Soon though, I was sliding my fingertip over the paper and placing a dot where my finger stopped, then sliding again to find where to place the next dot, and then connecting them. Not long after that, I was drawing only what I saw on the paper, what I call "unconceived drawing." I know that sounds like a simple explanation, but I truly disconnected my imagination and ego from the process and captured only what the paper showed me. The Command Screw is an example of the beginning and end of the process, since the screw was one of the first pictures I drew and the bridle and background were done with the unconceived technique. In this way, I was awed by what I helped bring to the material and have no doubt that even more power for good was brought with them. The Wild Cards discussed in this book will be available in a deck in the near future.

Using the Wild Cards, *does not* give you license to ignore your doctor or psychologist's orders, nor should you stop taking medications without their permission. Some of the approaches discussed in this book can cause physical symptoms, which may disappear after cleansing, but I strongly urge you to work with your medical practitioners so you're both on the same page when it comes to healing your body, mind, and spirit. Wild Card Therapy can be used in conjunction with conventional treatments, and should not reject them. Consult your physicians before using Wild Card Therapy if you have any medical concerns.

The methods in this book work *if* you're determined to be clean and whole. You can't simply give lip service and expect results. Unlike many spiritual teachings, I urge you to *use* your emotions. *Demand* to be clean. Get *angry* if something overlaps or clings to your personal space. Be *determined* to reject anything or anyone hindering your free will choice on your true pathway into the True United Destiny we all share.

While it's true that if your emotions control you they can cause trouble for yourself and those around you, when you control and use your emotions effectively, they become weapons of power capable of slicing through even the most atrophied crud, or the strongest bindings others have attempted to hinder you with. Without the emotional weapons born of your own heart, soul, and mind nothing in this book will work, but with the emotional at your disposal nothing can stand in your way (provided you don't attempt to hinder someone else).

Commit now to becoming clean and whole. This is a lifestyle change, and if you're not willing to commit to it, don't even start. Why? Because once you begin to strip away the layers which clog up the true you, what lies beneath *will* surface and demand attention. Whether you believe in past lives or not, your spirit is ancient and has experienced much since its birth from the True Creator's awareness. All that time must be taken into account in cleansing the self. So, I say again, if you aren't willing to make the lifestyle changes necessary to commit to cleansing your whole self, don't begin.

Whatever your religious beliefs, Wild Card Therapy can work for you, since beings beyond the material are doing most of the work. As long as you demand that only those who are appropriate act on the commands contained in this book, you need not worry about their names matching those of your religion. Those beings know their jobs regardless of the names people assign them. Focus your intent upon the job at hand, and have faith that those whose job it is to deal with those problems will act, as long as you do your part in wielding your strong desire for cleansing and growth.

However, I must also state that the beings mentioned in this book are real, not energies, and they work most efficiently when you accept them as being real. For example, a man we worked with refused to believe the Holy Spirit was a real being, insisting he was merely divine energies, and then becoming frustrated because his requests were not met with the same intensity others have experienced. It wasn't that the Holy Spirit was slacking off, but rather that he was being hindered in his work because of the man's beliefs. We can hinder those in spirit from helping us by setting up blocks that prevent them from doing their work to the fullest, even though they want to lend their aid.

Do not use the knowledge in this book to harm others. If you attempt to harm others, your Core Self and those beyond the material will rebound that wrongful use of power back on you and use the commands you uttered (silently or otherwise) as permission to cleanse your desire to harm or hinder others. Use this book only to heal and clean yourself and those who desire your help; beware of attempting to harm others or even cleanse them without permission. While a child seven years of age or younger may be cleansed without permission, I don't recommend cleansing children except under extreme circumstances. Any attempt to use this book and its knowledge wrongfully is not tolerated by the True Creator who granted this knowledge.

Realize that nothing is set in stone as far as the commands are concerned. Once you've learned these techniques, you may find they become less effective due to the intelligence of those you are attempting to clear. If they have been buried within you and surface only after you've cleared away several layers, those things have also been learning the techniques. You may find many who, once coming to the surface, are eager to be gone and will thank you for recognizing and freeing them; others may be stubborn and have thought up ways to refuse the commands. If they refuse, modify the commands. How? Use your instinct. Feel what it is they are using to hinder the commands and shift the wording slightly. For example, "See those whom you love and trust waiting to take you home to the light," may evolve into, "See those who are laughing at you for overlapping me because they are claiming the place where you are supposed to be." Use your instincts to feel the truth of what to say and do, whether these things overlap you or are clinging outside. Trust yourself and use these techniques as base lines in evolving powerful techniques of your own, but only after you have cleared using the basic commands.

If you find that you stir up things which are hard to handle, call on "the appropriate part of Aunt" to come and deal with it or find us on the website below. I'm not saying this as an ego thing, but as an approach that works. Many people have called on the appropriate part of me to help, and have found I'm quickly there to lend aid, even though my conscious mind is unaware of it. When you think of it, it's not so far fetched, since the greater part of us is spirit, too vast to squeeze into the material body.

Aunt T'

Throughout this book, things may be stirred simply by reading a certain section. Your feelings may vary from anger, frustration, or fear to that of betrayal. You may not be able to clearly identify what is causing these feelings. Aunt T' Pathfinder brought this knowledge into the material, and encourages you to send to her all causing the feelings stirred as a result. You need not worrying about harming her, as she is experienced in dealing with all sent to her, and in fact it aids her personal cleansing. Note though, while this will not harm Aunt T', it can cause harm and chaos to others, so please ensure your thought intent in sending is to her, and her only, in all ways appropriate.

Finally, we hope you will allow the information shared in this book to assist you in finding your true self and true pathway. The journey in finding yourself is an empowering and joyous one. You will be amazed to see and feel your strength and the bright shining light within. Please enjoy this book. If you would like to share your successes or have questions, we can be reached at healingmindandspirit@hotmail.com.

Gail Marie

Chapter 1:
Healing

What is Healing?

GAIL MARIE: Once you have made the decision to pursue personal growth or personal healing, cleansing your energy and parts of the self (see Chapter 2) is an extremely important part of that process. Cleansing, by definition, is the process of purifying, or for our purposes, removing all that is not truly you. This gives you back control of yourself and your healing.

Healing is done in layers. A good analogy is to relate it to an onion, in that you need to peel the layers from an onion to get to the core.

AUNT T': Continuing with the onion analogy, once you've removed the outside layer, you may feel wonderful for a while and believe you are finished with cleansing, but then the next layer begins to smell as what's buried there begins to surface and cause trouble. How long it takes you to get through the layers of the "onion" depends on how may lifetimes you've lived and how much karma has been accumulated. Remember that even karma credit is attached to someone holding the debit end, so all aspects of it must be dealt with. Leaving the onion analogy behind, the closer you get to the core of yourself, the lighter and stronger you'll feel. The parts of you that have been suppressed by the weight of what did not belong will begin to surface. You are the focus, the awareness, which was born from the True Creator's own awareness in the first nanoseconds of time. Don't give up after just a few cleansing sessions, because the end result is awesome as you reclaim the "You" who God, the True Creator, birthed you to become.

GM: For many, healing seems like a daunting task, one that can create fear of having to deal with buried or unresolved issues. Something important to remember is that *issues or feelings that are hindering you (from your personal growth, healing, and development) can only hurt* *you when they are not healed*. You will encounter times in your healing when you feel like giving up, like it's not working. Take those times as clues that releasing is needed. Once you remove one layer, you'll feel great, until the next layer surfaces for healing. Use the time between layers to motivate you to keep going. Each time you release, you'll feel better and that you are progressing. The more you remove, the less baggage you have to drag you down or hinder you.

Unbeknownst to many, we are very complex creatures. Many parts of the self are identified in this book. What's important in learning about them, is not remembering the individual parts, but recognizing them as places needing to be healed and cleansed. We are not only affected by things in the material world, but in other realms as well. This chapter focuses on things that can affect our healing and cleansing in this and other realms. Chapter 2 provides the actual steps in cleansing using Wild Cards.

Because we are so complex, releasing things can stir up other things hiding beneath or behind what you are releasing, so it's important if you are releasing and still not feeling your true self, that you repeat the cleansing process until you feel the true you. Wild Card Therapy calls on you to take control of your healing and responsibility for your emotions. Once past situations have been healed, it's up to you to decide how you want to deal with future situations. You can choose to continue to respond to them as you always have, or with the new perspective you've realized through healing. Relying on and trusting your knowledge can accomplish this. Throughout the book, you will be asked questions and told to trust your first thought as the appropriate answer. When hearing that first thought, ensure that it's coming from the center of your head. If it isn't, and you know it isn't you, or you receive negative answers, then call on Archangel Michael to clear all hindering you from hearing the appropriate part of yourself.

When using the Wild Cards, you will similarly be asked to trust your instinct and use the cards you feel are appropriate or drawn to.

Before proceeding with an explanation of the importance and process of cleansing, it's important to have an understanding of the following terms.

Light, Energy, Power

AT': Light, energy, and power are all born from the True Creator, but are refined as they flow into the inner regions of existence where we reside. Scientists say that everything is shaped from energy; it's true, since all the refining and condensing through gravity creates this material realm of ours. If you were to step outside the material and look back at it, you would see this, but since we are within material bodies, we are often blind to this fact. Light is also energy, less refined and yet more focused, because to call on any form of light is to call upon the True Creator's awareness of our needs. As for power, it can be either light or energy, since it is the mind that gives it form and emotions that refine it with our intent.

So, which is more powerful, light or energy? It depends on the intent behind their use and how much refining has occurred before they are used. White light is refined through the Spirit Realms and under the command of the Christed One and others who work on the positive side of balance. Of course, the opposite is true for dark light, used by those on the negative side of balance, while those in the center wield any light they believe is needed to maintain balance. Some people flinch away from using negative energy, having been taught that it is evil, but this is a hindrance to understanding wholeness of the self. Negative energy is as essential to being whole as positive energy is, and to deprive ourselves of one or the other hinders our growth, causing us to repeat lessons to teach us how to use them for the good of self and all.

GM: A familiar example of the benefit of negative energy is its ability to make us aware of things surfacing, giving us a nudge to look at what's causing the feeling and pushing us toward healing. Frustration with the world around us is also a clue that we need to deal with something within.

AT': Whichever you use, remember this: even if you use only positive energies, rebounding can occur if they are wrongfully used or used on someone who rejects them. So, which is more powerful? That which is used appropriately.

Core energies are your birthright from the True Creator and they rise from the center of your being, feeding you directly from the True Creator. They come from within, not outside, and as such cannot be bound or warped by anyone but your Core Self. Any energy or light sent to you from outside can be warped by another's intent, even if that intent is good and honorable, since he or she can only guess at what you truly need at that point on your pathway. Better for another to help you learn to access your own core energies than to warp you by sending you something which may not be compatible with your Core Self's intent.

GM: The pure light is unrefined light coming straight from God, the True Creator. It is the most powerful form of light you can use and is the source of unconditional love. The quicksilver is antiquity's martyred blood condensed since the beginning of time and ignited by the pure light sword of Archangel Michael. God melded the quicksilver with the pure light to create the Wild Cards and other spiritual tools that help cleanse and heal humanity and other life in the material world and beyond.

The pure light quicksilver has sprouted fountains that are used alone or in conjunction with the blood of Jesus Christ to cleanse people inside and out. It is most intense in spirit and has been known to heal some of the wildest spirits and return them to the light of the True Creator, but even in the flesh it can be felt like a refreshing spring rain. To feel the pure light quicksilver, follow these steps.

1. Visualize a large fountain, with a round pool at its base and a plain center that draws up water and releases it to flow down and around.
2. Call upon Archangel Michael and ask him to transform your visualization of the fountain's water into the pure light quicksilver.
3. Once he tells you it has been done, step into the fountain and feel the quicksilver flowing down upon you, or lie in it and allow it to soak into you, washing you clean.

Inner Core Self

AT': I have noticed some confusion about what the inner core is. Many people I speak with think it's their higher self, but it isn't. The Core Self is that part of you which sprouts all the other parts of yourself. Like an acorn that sprouts a mighty oak tree, some parts of you grow upward into the light, while other parts grow inward to nourish you with your roots. Appendix 3 lists the parts of you that sprout from the core. Note that the core is not listed among them, since it is not subject to growth, being greater than all the other parts already. Chapter 7 has a section on the regions within you and what the core holds, as well as an exercise for stripping away false cores. In Chapter 8 there's an exercise for reclaiming your Ivory Tower (see cover) and Control Room. I recommend that you do those only after you have begun to feel secure in the cleansing exercises featured in earlier chapters.

Personal Shields

GM: Our personal shields are created of pure light from our energy and are used for the protection of our whole being. It is extremely important to have and keep your shields strong to prevent the clinging and pocketing of spirits. There are a number of energies, objects and beings that must be cleansed from our personal space to allow us to begin the healing process. (See Appendix 5.)

AT': Personal shields are born from your Core Self and shaped from the pure light and your own core energies. This ensures that they are always pure and commanded by you alone. When dealing with any being with awareness, it's appropriate for you to call upon that individual's core energies and to wrap them tightly, ensuring the beings of light can tell the difference between you and it. In establishing your shields, trust your Core Self and personal shields to know what to allow and what to reject, since your core knows what is appropriate to your true pathway at any given point.

Overlapping

GM: When you are overlapped, you have something clinging to or pocketing inside your personal shields.

AT': When people use the term "possession" they are speaking of the most intense form of overlapping, which is rare and only occurs when the host is weakened or willingly gives up control of his or her body to the being overlapping it. Usually, those who overlap a host can do little more than whisper disruptive thoughts or cause medically puzzling pain.

Using myself as an example, I was thirty-eight years old before I knew what a silent mind was. I had been overlapped by many disruptive beings my entire life and it was only after my first hypnotherapy session that my mind was silent. That silence didn't last long because the layers of beings beneath those removed began to surface, but I knew by then what they were and began to evolve the tools and commands in this book to deal with them. I didn't want others to experience the pain of such beings fighting to remain, and so the removal techniques in this book do so without harm to either the one overlapped or those who are being removed.

No matter the strength of the being overlapping an individual, they do not belong. This book gives you the tools to remove them and reclaim your personal space.

Symbionts

AT': Symbionts are those microorganisms that live within and on us to keep us healthy and balanced. Some exist in your spirit, as well as your body, such as the mitochondria. Mitochondria are found in every cell of your body, given to you by your birth mother, but the united mind within them comes with you from spirit. I say "united mind" because they have their own awareness, which united as a single entity, you can communicate with. Your mitochondrial mind is one of the best friends and guides you have. It's your life-long companion and, at times when your own awareness is disabled for some reason, it can take over as your automatic pilot. You speak to your mitochondria through the base of your brain, where the brain stem comes from your neck and joins the brain. It's centered there, so if you ask it a question and hear an answer either to the left or right, then you have contacted another symbiont united mind, of which you have three others. The left-of-center voice, at the base of your brain, is that of the symbionts who interact with the analytical side of your brain. The voice right of center, at the base, is that of the symbionts who interact with the spiritual and creative side of the brain. The fourth voice is deeper, heard in the throat area, and is entwined with your lymphatic, or immune, system.

To communicate with your symbionts, simply clear your mind, focus on them, ask them to identify themselves, then listen for the answer. Note where the answering voice comes from. Your mitochondrial united mind will give you a name, and that name will always be of the opposite gender from yours, offering a yin-yang type of balance. The other three (analytical, spiritual, lymphatic) are always the same gender as you are physically, since they don't follow you beyond the flesh, nor do they see themselves as having a name beyond your own. If you receive answers from your symbionts that contradict what I've stated here, there's interference and you need to do the cleansing techniques found in the following chapters to clear the way before trying again.

GM: The guide I work with is that of my mitochondrial mind. In working with him, I am confident that, when questioning and accessing knowledge, I haven't been hindered or influenced by outsiders.

Merged Spirits

GM: A merged spirit is one that has been with you for many lives and has been able to merge their energy with yours, making it difficult to distinguish between what is truly you and what is the other spirit. In order to distinguish between what is truly you or another, you can call on your spirit mate to identify what is truly you. Spirit mates are not always soul mates, although they can be. Many spirit mates are never born into flesh, remaining pure spirit to aid us from the light if necessary. Soul mates, in general, are those we have incarnated with many times and have grown closest to within our soul group.

AT': Merged spirits are a rare thing, but troublesome. I know. I myself was affected by a merged spirit who was with me from my first lifetime until 1993, when she was finally identified and removed. She had been clinging to the embryo prepared for me, but since she didn't have permission to take that body, she clung to it and to me once I finally claimed it. Having never been in flesh, I had no idea that the way she made me feel was not normal. In the years since her removal, I have found Awareness, Layer, Pseudo-self children (ALPs) of her, which the Holy Spirit dealt with after my spirit mates identified the difference between them and me.

I have also come to understand that many of the things I did and said over my sixty-eight lifetimes was her and not me. Although the memories are mine, the karma created by those events belongs to her. I have also found atrophied pieces of me which died from being choked off from the rest of me by her presence and had to be cleansed away, recycled as crud or as ALPs. There were also parts of me so contaminated by her, that they were no longer me, and I had to deliberately calve them away and deliver them to the Holy Spirit to be born separately from me when their time is appropriate.

Along with all the above, the problem with the merged spirit is that it calved away ALPs during all of those lifetimes and even now, years after having removed the parent awareness, I continue to come upon ALPs of her. The number of ALPs depends on how many years or lifetimes the merged spirit overlapped you. In my case, I have sixty-eight lifetimes worth of her ALPs to find and remove. They're easy enough to remove once they stir and are identified. Just wrap them in the pure light quicksilver and ask the Holy Spirit to gather them in and deal with them appropriately.

The Ivy, The Vines, The Creator's Milk

GM: The ivy is a wonderful tool created to help us heal. The ivy was created to help those who pass on to cleanse, removing all the baggage created in material lifetimes. The wonderful thing is that we in the material world are also able to access it just by visualizing it and calling it to us. It will give you a relaxed, calm, and peaceful feeling. I do this visualization for myself every night before I fall asleep. You will notice the ivy will wrap around you wherever it is appropriate. Personally, I'm not able to see it, but I can feel it pulsating where it's wrapping. If at any time the ivy gives you a choking feeling, it is a sign that it requires more help in the cleansing process. Following the cleansing commands in the next chapter will help to deal with whatever the ivy has identified.

Wrapped in and around the ivy is a vine. The flowers blooming on this vine are white and bell shaped. When called upon, the flowers on the vine will create a vacuum suction to vacuum up all those things hindering self-love. Those things which require your conscious attention and release will be held by the flowers of the vine, until appropriate release can be completed. In my experience using the vine with others, we have been able to identify cycles, so further focus can be placed on those particular areas for release.

Also, at the gates of the garden of light, you have access to the Creator's milk. The job of this milk is to help clear away those extra stubborn things hindering the healing and growth processes.

All are fantastic tools that can help you find and identify hindrances to your healing and growth and can be used any time you feel the need by simply calling on them and allowing them to do their jobs.

AT': I see the ivy and vine mentioned above as being on the right-hand side of Saint Peter's Gate as you approach it. On the left are two more vines. The ivy is tuned to the mitochondria within you, and the vine is tuned to the spiritual and creative symbionts in the right side of your brain. The two on the left of the gate are for the other two symbiotic systems of your body.

Nearest to the center is the vine tuned to the analytical side of your brain and it has no leaves. Instead, its pale blue flowers grow from the vine's trunk and vanish as the side branches begin to grow. These side branches grow in a curly spiral and when called on they unwind and grasp the thought patterns hindering your growth. Once these thought patterns have been contained by the vine, they are broken down and vacuumed out through the vine's tip.

The other vine works with the lymphatic system's symbionts to add strength to your immune system. This vine has pale pink flowers that also grow on the stem of the vine and last only long enough to sprout multiple vines that grow in a tangled mass. When called on, this mass reaches out to all parts of your lymphatic system to cleanse it so it can become more efficient at protecting you. If there is need, it will also travel throughout your body to help fight off invaders. Know that for this vine to be effective, it has to be part of your true pathway to be healed, so double-check with your Spirit Guides to see if it is appropriate.

The roots of the vines and the ivy are sunk deep into the stream of the Creator's milk, which flows from the garden. The source of the Creator's milk is the True Creator's unconditional love, surfacing through a rocky alcove that exists beneath Christ's tower and flowing throughout the garden of light, through the gate and outward to all places of existence.

Awareness, Layer, Pseudo-self Children (ALPs)

GM: Awareness, layer children (ALs) were at one time part of us, but are no longer. They are created daily. More traumatic times in our lives can create ALs that affect us more than the day to day ones we create. If you think of your energy as the whole, an AL is a piece of that whole which has been fractured off. When they are fractured off, in most cases, they cling to your shields and can affect you by continually stirring up the emotions you felt when they were created. ALs can be found in any of our layers.

Pseudo-self Children (Ps) are similar to AL children, in that they used to be part of us. The difference between the two is where they are found. With Ps, a part of them is found in all of our layers and all the pieces join together to make a whole.

AT': It is important to note that ALs are confined to an individual layer, but are created in sibling groups within each of our layers. This means that when you find one, there will be others, so it's important to clear them from all your layers, regardless of whether or not you have identified them individually. The Holy Spirit can see the sibling groups even if you can't. If you consider yourself a first-generation child born from the Creator, your ALPs are second generation, the Creator's grandchildren.

As Gail Marie said, they tend to cling to the parent awareness when they calve away, but there are circumstances in which they are found elsewhere. One of these circumstances is when the trauma is so great, they flee outward, in which case they tend to wrap time around themselves and create a pocket of warped time (see Appendix 9). Here, they attempt to escape from the trauma either by rejecting it completely or by attempting to change the ending. The other circumstance is when the parent is overlapping another being's personal space when the ALP is formed. When the parent is removed, the child stays behind, but must be identified and rejected. In either case, the Holy Spirit is needed to deal with them.

GM: There is also an opportunity in which a dominant ALP may cause you to feel that you have lost time or can't remember what you've done. You might notice that your behavior has been unlike your normal behavior. If you were to ask, "Am I the true owner of this body?" you might find a *No* answer popping into your head. This is a clue that an ALP is causing the behavior. If you find this is the case, release your ALP to the Holy Spirit and he will deal with that child.

I've also worked on cases where the person isn't aware that an ALP is at the surface. As an outsider looking in, you may not be able to notice in others when an ALP is surfacing because the person won't look different and their voice will be the same, but there are subtle clues like the words or the mood of the person won't seem normal for them.

An example of an ALP at the surface, which I experienced with someone, occurred when they described themselves as dirty, ashamed and not worthy of the guidance I was giving them. Knowing this person quite well, I knew this wasn't her true self talking, and I asked the one I was talking with to call on the Holy Spirit to see if she could go with Him to heal. Of course the answer was *Yes* and she described to me what happened just before she went with Him. She described Him touching her hand and all the darkness and dirtiness she felt was transmuted into pure white, releasing those feelings of shame and unworthiness.

Another example of a more common ALP came from a woman who had been in a car accident years before. Currently, she was taking driving lessons, wasn't able to focus, and was feeling fear and disappointment with her progress. I asked her to identify the feelings she'd had at the time of the accident and we released those feelings. We then released her ALPs related to that incident. I spoke with her a few days later and she was amazed at how well she was doing and how the feelings she had previously experienced earlier in her driving lessons were gone.

Emotion Seeds, Memory Pods, Shadow Sheets

GM: Emotion seeds, memory pods and shadow sheets are all energy residues born of intense emotions. Depending on the intensity of the emotion, incident or issue, ALPs can be created simultaneously. Any of these energy residues can hide ALPs and may have karmic ties too. Beings that require cleansing can also hide in and around emotion seeds, memory pods or shadow sheets. If intense or layered enough, they can be blocked off from the rest of your being resulting in atrophy, in a sense dying and becoming removed from you. Archangels Michael and Raphael are responsible for dealing with any energy or being hiding in or between any of our layers or overlapping us.

AT': As an example, I take something from my own life. It involves an incident from my childhood, when I was about a year and a half old. My Father molested me, hurting me in that private place and then comforting me afterwards, telling me he was sorry and how much he loved me. In those moments, a memory pod was created to bind the incident, emotion seeds were born to contain the emotions, and a shadow sheet wrapped me to buffer the pain of my flesh. These three things remained with me years after the incident, irritated by the ALPs which were created at the same time, and their combination left me weak and open to attachments and overlapping by many dark, wild beings over the years. Although this memory was the most dominant from my childhood, I was unable to completely heal until all the components were dealt with, including the "crud" that had settled into the cracks between these energies and the true me over the years. Now, looking back on the clean memory of that time, I can see it clearly and without pain or fear. Since my Father died soon after I began school, I had to release the karmic ties, forgiving him, soul to soul. Although that sounds like a complex thing to do, once identified, these things can all be dealt with simultaneously by asking Archangel Michael and others to help you release and cleanse yourself, while calling upon your own core energies to rise up and push them out from the inside.

I used the above example to show you that anything can be forgiven and healed if you have the strength to look at it clearly and understand that growth can only be achieved by dealing with the past and loving who you are now.

Message Bubbles

GM: Message bubbles pass communication from one part of us to another, but once their use is fulfilled, if they don't dissolve, they become a problematic energy residue that needs to be dealt with. Message bubbles can also be seen as false beings, as in a pod of emotion or energy that flows from one part of us to another. If undissolved, they gain weight outside us and appear as whom we expect them to. These false beings created through message bubbles have no thought or emotion of their own, instead being driven by all we project into them. Warping occurs through this projection of our thoughts and emotions onto others, believing them to be the spirit they are mirroring. These situations are not appropriate and the Archangel Azrael can be called upon to deal with all found mimicking a spirit.

Thought Clusters

GM: Thought clusters surface when an experience or event in this life is similar to one in a past life. It can create confusion and block off choices in this life. Also considered an energy residue, thought clusters need to be dealt with appropriately.

Paradox Directional Selves (PDSs)

GM: The PDS (see Appendix 4) is similar to an ALP, but in this case, is both male and female, and a part of the self. When working appropriately, the role of the PDS is to help us maintain balance and enable us to follow our True Pathways into the First Dream (see Appendix 11). When out of balance, PDSs can cause a variety of problems. PDSs are a necessary part of the self and must be dealt with firmly, but gently, and with compassion.

Grounding

GM: Another form of protection that can be used in conjunction with your personal shields is grounding. Grounding allows us to communicate with spirits of higher vibrations, while remaining tied to the earth plane, rather than feeling lightheaded or floating.

A permanent way to ground is to call on your Core Self, and picture a root growing from your core down into the ground. See an answering root coming from the planet's core reaching towards the root growing from you. As they grow together, watch them become a single strong root, and feel the Earth's nourishing energies flowing up into you. Now call on your Core Self and symbionts to rebalance your energy appropriately. The root growing from you should be a single healthy strand. If it isn't, ask Archangel Michael to deal appropriately with all hindering this. This grounding will remain for as long as you are in flesh, but will fall away once you leave your flesh behind.

AT': It must also be noted that if you are visual and see more than one root coming from your Core Self to reach the planet's core, then a cleansing must be done to remove those beings whose roots are reaching down along with your own. Each person has only one anchoring root, so the presence of others is a clue that cleansing is required.

Pseudo-Nephilim

GM: The pseudo-nephilim are described in Enoch's book as well as the book of Genesis in the Bible. They are fathered by angels and mothered by human women. The 200 or so pseudo-Nephilim were cursed by the regional godling as evil and left wandering the earth. They have been found overlapping people's personal space, where they hide, afraid of discovery. Once their siblings in the light are called upon to speak with them, they learn the curse has been removed, and they are free to go to the light. They will go willingly and in my experience, return to help protect us as requested.

What is Being Cleansed and Why is it Important to Cleanse Our Energy?

GM: To understand why cleansing is important, we need an understanding of what energies can affect us. Humans are complex and have lived many lives, however, cleansing energy is a new concept. To heal ourselves, we need to ensure that it is only us we are dealing with. Anything that is not truly us, we can't heal. By cleansing your energy, you ensure that nothing will hinder your growth, development, and healing.

At some point in our past or present lives, we've had other energies, objects, or beings overlapping our space (see Appendix 1). These intrusions influence our thoughts, emotions, and actions. In most cases, these things that cling to us don't control our actions, unless we allow them to.

Have you ever had trouble quieting your mind? Have you ever had thoughts that just didn't seem like you? Have you ever acted and wondered, "Why did I do that?" If you answered yes to any of these questions, then further investigation is required to understand whether or not you are being affected by something other than the true you. An overlapping object, energy, or being is not the same as a merged spirit.

To understand overlapping, a balloon is a good analogy. A balloon full of air represents our personal shields at full strength. If you tried to put your finger through the balloon, the strength of the air inside it would prevent your finger from reaching the middle. It wouldn't allow anything to cling to it because a balloon offers nothing to hold onto. A balloon half full of air represents your shields when they are weakened. Now your finger can be pushed into the balloon's center without resistance. You can also grab the side of the balloon and cling to it easily. If your finger represents a spirit, energy, or object, and the balloon represents your true self, you can understand how we can be effected by them. While these intrusions don't break through your shields, through pocketing in your defenses, they can get close enough to your center to affect you.

AT': Know that *nothing* can penetrate the core of your being, no matter how close they come. However, they can stand between our conscious mind and our core, or create "things" which hinder us from reaching our real core, tricking us into believing we are there when we are not.

GM: To deal with any energy, object, or being overlapping us, we call on Archangel Michael who, in conjunction with the appropriate Wild Cards, is responsible for dealing with them.

The next part of cleansing is to release ALPs. These children cling to us, but are no longer a part of us, so we can never truly heal them. For example, if you were in a car accident, you'd create one or more ALPs at that moment. You may feel you've healed from the accident, but when you get back into a car or other vehicle, all those feelings and thoughts you experienced during the accident come rushing back. This is an example of an ALP clinging and affecting you. No matter how many emotional releases or how much healing you do related to the accident, you won't be able to heal completely until you release those ALPs.

Remember when you are cleansing that it is not a one-time process. The baggage we carry wasn't created in a short time, so the healing required isn't short term. You will, however, start to notice a difference fairly quickly, and that should encourage you to continue the process. When we use the commands to cleanse, we are cleansed appropriately, but can only deal with what is at the surface or in the open. To reach those hidden things, we need to cleanse regularly. As you become more familiar with the true you, you'll begin to know when something is intruding and how to deal with it appropriately.

AT': Once you've removed several layers of what overlaps you, you may feel you are not yourself, or that you don't feel as you used to, and yet you are calmer and better able to deal with the world around you. This is because you are finally able to feel your true self, rather than those things that have been overlapping you. Remember that before the cleansing, you were feeling only a small part of yourself, buried by all the "crud" and others overlapping your personal space. Once you are cleansed, you're bound to feel different.

Chapter 2:
The Cleansing Process

Part I: Standard Cleansing

GM: What follows is an easy and effective standard cleansing that can be done regularly. When you're done, you'll find a more in-depth cleansing that reaches deeper into the self in Part II.

Standard Cleansing Process

1. Before you begin, request that Archangel Michael bind, with pure light quicksilver and appropriate core energies, any energy, object, or being that is inappropriate to your self. This will ensure that the spirit or energy being removed won't be able to migrate into someone else and that it will receive the appropriate healing.

2. Now say silently or aloud, "I reject any energy, object, or being not truly me or mine, and I ask my spirit mate to identify what is truly me, and I call on Archangel Michael to deal appropriately with that which is not truly me."

3. Pay attention to how you are feeling. Is your head feeling dizzy, fuzzy, foggy? Do you have any heaviness anywhere in your body? The response from people is very individual, and in some cases, you may feel very tired or physically uncomfortable. Whatever you feel is appropriate, but it isn't appropriate for it to remain, so do not accept it. Continue rejecting these feelings until you feel totally clear.

4. If any of the above feelings continue, repeat step 2.

5. Continue to reject these feelings until you feel light and clear-headed.

6. If you find you still aren't clear-headed, or feel like something is preventing whatever is overlapping you from leaving, you need to deal with it. There are a number of things that could be affecting you, for instance, a curse, spell, or vow (see Appendix 1) may have been placed on you either in this lifetime or in past lives. See section below on "Removal of Curse, Vow, or Spell" for instructions on how to release it.

7. If, after using these releases, you find you're *still* not clear-headed and/or feel heaviness, proceed to a deep cleansing using the Wilds Cards by calling on all appropriate to activate.

8. Once the spirit or energy has been removed, ask your core energies to fill all the emptied spaces. This will ensure that nothing else occupies them.

9. After completing the above process, the last step is to wrap all the pain, hurt, anger, or other negative emotions with pure light and send it to the True Creator to be dealt with appropriately. If at any time you feel pain, tingling, or any other sensation that wasn't there when you started, that's a clue to focus on sending it and its cause to the True Creator. There need not be any fear of overloading the True Creator; what is sent is ensured of healing and recycling in the pure light. When you do this, say silently or aloud, "I reject all that is hindering me from finding and walking my true pathway and release it all, including karma and karmic ties."

Throughout your cleansing and healing process, it's important to call on your Inner Core to rise up and strengthen you, and fill vacated areas with the pure light quicksilver and appropriate core energies. We've also found that visualizing a "safe place" in your mind while undergoing this process is very effective in helping us to relax and continue healing without fear or outside influences. I go to a place I refer to as "my high spot," a place high above the material world. For example, I might visualize climbing a spiral staircase to the top of a high building to begin my healing work.

AT': A "safe place" is any place you can visualize where you feel safe and protected from that which is not you. Visualize it as being surrounded by pure light that nothing can get through unless you consciously allow it to. By imagining this place as a building, and the building as being your body, you have the option of using it to explore in two different directions, inwardly or outwardly. By visualizing a trap door at the highest point, you can open that door and descend into your own being to cleanse or explore your inner layers, or other aspects of your inner self. From the highest point of the building, you also have the option of projecting your spirit outward towards the garden of light or anywhere else you have permission to explore. Spirit projection is not astral travel, since your soul stays where it is; in spirit projection, we tap into our spirit, which extends beyond our flesh body. When you go outward, it's always a good idea to have your Spirit Guides and Guardian Angels accompany you to ensure your safety and open the way for you.

Releasing Awareness, Layer, and Pseudo-self Children (ALPs)

GM: To release awareness, layer, and pseudo-self children, say, "I wrap any and all ALPs in pure light quicksilver and their own core energies, as I call on the Holy Spirit to deal with them all appropriately. If there are any which have not fully broken away from me, I also wrap them in the pure light quicksilver and their core energies, as I ask that Archangel Michael and his legions wield their weapons of pure light and slice them free from me, gathering in anyone who is hiding between them and me as the Holy Spirit takes them as soon as they are free. Thank you."

AT': Another simple method of removing ALPs, called the ALP mirrors, has evolved over time, because some people have trouble letting them go, thinking the ALPs are still part of themselves.

1. Visualize three beautifully framed, full-length mirrors made of titanium standing just millimeters away from you. The one on the right is for your ALPs; the one in the center is for the ALPs of intruders or those who have overlapped you; and the one on the left is for ALP clumps and ALPs from other time rounds (see Appendix 12). Know that the Holy Spirit is on the other side of these mirrors waiting to guide all the ALPs to their appropriate places, where they will be loved and cared for. At the top of each mirror is a flashing neon sign, which will attract the ALPs. Also, your Core Self will automatically fill in all emptied areas and Archangel Michael will automatically be granted permission to cleanse anything that was between the ALPs and yourself.
2. To activate the mirrors, simply remark on how pretty the mirrors are, either aloud or silently. The ALPs will usually begin leaving on

their own. If they don't, tell them how much love and joy is awaiting them, and ask that they see this in the mirrors. If they still don't leave, it may be because they're afraid you will be harmed by a memory they are suppressing. If this is the case, tell them that you've grown beyond who you were when that memory was formed, and that you are harmed more by not dealing with the memory than you would be by their releasing it and allowing you to deal with it.

3.   If for any reason your mirrors stop working, ask that the old mirrors be recycled and then repeat the above steps to create new ones.

GM: In cases where you're not sure if an ALP is present, call on the Holy Spirit. Confirm that you are speaking with the Holy Spirit, then ask him if you can go with him to heal. Take your first thought as his answer; if the answer is *Yes*, then it is an awareness child at the surface. If the answer is *No*, then you can be assured that it is you, the true owner of the body, in control. In cases of pseudo-self children, it's easier to release them if you call on the ivy for assistance.

We've noticed that with dominant ALPs there can be a "captain," a leader for others. My discovery of this was an interesting experience. I was working with a child releasing her ALPs. I asked her to ask the Holy Spirit if she could go with Him to heal. The answer she got was *Yes*. I asked her to go and she said yes, but then she started laughing uncontrollably. I asked if she could see anything leaving, and she said yes, but the particular ALP that was dominant at the surface hadn't gone yet. When I asked her to describe what she was seeing, she described a boat with many on it dancing and laughing. Within a few minutes of her seeing this, she saw herself and others following the Holy Spirit through a musical forest and then they were gone. The laughing was a delay tactic from the dominant ALP, the "captain." The dominant one wasn't going to leave until all the others within its "group" were identified and with the Holy Spirit.

AT': When removing ALPs, also remember to ask the Holy Spirit to take all which belong to other awarenesses as well. You need both your own and those calved away from intruders to be taken from you, since no one has a right to be in your personal space except yourself and the appropriate symbionts needed to keep you balanced and healthy. So, wrap *all* ALPs in the pure light quicksilver and core energies, both yours and those belonging to others, then push them all outside yourself and hand them over to the Holy Spirit or allow them to go through your ALP mirrors.

When you come upon stubborn kids who refuse to leave with the Holy Spirit, they could be clinging for several reasons. Maybe they haven't fully fractured away from you; you need to consciously demand that they do so. There could also be tendrils of them attached; they're clinging hard to parts of you, to past events, energy objects, or perhaps waiting for something to occur before completely breaking away. Where there are tendrils, you must pull up each one individually to see what it is and deal with it accordingly through the cleansing techniques and tools listed throughout the book, according to what you find at the end of each individual tendril.

The normal procedure for dealing with these more difficult ALPs is to ask the Holy Spirit to be gentle, and ensure the child isn't fractured into more pieces than it already is. The child might have awareness, layer children of its own that are clinging to both it and you. Call upon the Holy Spirit to check on this and deal with *all* generations of children appropriately. There are very few second-generation children who have a right to interact in our realms of existence, and no third- or later generations should be here. This place was created for us, for the True Creator's first generation, and so the Holy Spirit takes all others to realms of light where they are prepared for the future, a future that awaits us all after the First Dream is manifest.

If you undertake all the above, and the child still doesn't budge, perhaps the child is awaiting some future event before breaking away. Here's an example of how I dealt with one such child. First, I checked to make sure all its siblings had been removed, which they had, and then I called upon the pure light quicksilver to shape gauze bandages in which I completely wrapped the child. This revealed several tendrils connecting the child to me. These tendrils were a mixture of things. One carried memories from the time of the child's creation when I was in the third grade; there was also an atrophied piece of me, energy objects, a fragment of an alien implant (most of which had already been found and removed), as well as pieces of me that were still active and needed. I removed all the tendrils except for those parts of me I was still using, and had drawn the child outside my personal shields, but she was still clinging hard. I asked the Holy Spirit to make sure there were no fragments of children within her, or even intruders who might be helping her cling to me, but she was clean. Finally, all that was left were those parts of me that I was using, parts that would eventually belong to her once I'd grown farther along my true pathway. Since I could still feel the child, even though she was out beyond my shields, I knew she needed to go, and the only way I could get rid of her was to get rid of those pieces of me she was clinging to. What I finally did was call upon those parts of me beneath the ones she was clinging to, consciously demanding that those parts copy what she was clinging to so she could take the originals without causing me harm. This worked and she finally left, but the parts that were copies of the originals needed time to adjust, and I found I had headaches for a while after this work. The headaches were worth it since I was freed from the child.

Releasing Body Energy Residue

GM: Next on our list of releases is dealing with body energy residue, consisting of emotion seeds, memory pods, shadow sheets, thought clusters, and message bubbles. To release these, say, "Archangel Raphael, please clear away all body energy residue, and Archangel Michael please deal with all else hidden in and around these which is not me." Next, overflow yourself in pure light and your core energies, filling all vacated areas.

Removal of Curse, Vow, or Spell

GM: To remove a curse, false vow, or spell, and all other wrongful uses of power, refer to the list in Appendix 1 and repeat the following: "I reject all curses, spells, false vows, and all wrongful uses of power placed on me and all relatives, including those married into the family (this lifetime and all past, present, and future lifetimes and time rounds) including those I may have placed on others. I acknowledge that no one or nothing has the right to hinder free will choice or my true pathway whether they be of the light, dark, or balance, and I call upon Archangel Michael and the Holy Spirit to deal with all hindering me in this manner.

AT': If these wrongful uses of power are being sent by someone in the flesh, you need to reject their right to bind you with such things. Call on your personal shields to reject them, and the pure light quicksilver to transmute and rebound those powers. When rebounding wrongful power, intermix it with unconditional love so that the one sending the wrongful power can be healed (having given up free will choice to reject cleansing when they attacked you). Besides, if you don't mix it with unconditional love, the rebound effect can be quite violent, something I learned when I tried rebounding as I'd been told to do in my youth (and have never done since).

As an example, I'll tell you of a man I worked with near the beginning of my journey to understanding these things. We were in the same art department, but different rooms. My job was to check what he sent me to make sure it was correct before forwarding it to the next step in the process, but one particular day, I found several mistakes and had to send it back to him. He became angry, and although he didn't say anything aloud, he was cursing me in his mind. I knew this because I felt wave after wave of anger coming from him and striking my shields. I rejected his right to attack me in such a way, and commanded the energies be rebounded to him, as I had always heard I should do. Within minutes, he became very chaotic and was verbally striking out at everyone around him, although his attention had turned away from me. In shock, I called upon Archangel Michael to transmute the energies and drain them away into the pure light so they would harm no one. So I learned that when you rebound energy, always transmute it with unconditional love so no one is harmed.

Transmuting wrongful uses of power with unconditional love before they are rebounded, also opens the attacker to cleansing those parts of the self which are attacking. This is the only time free will is overridden regarding cleansing. Remember this: if you're going to attack someone, verbally or psychically, you give up your choice to refuse cleansing. If you don't wish to be cleansed against your will, then don't attack others.

Free Will Versus Curses and Such

GM: In relation to our free will, it's important to know that there's opportunity for others to affect it without our knowledge. The best way to protect yourself is by being aware and knowledgeable, so you can use the releases in this book to remove these threats and shield yourself.

Thought energy is very powerful whether used for your highest good or used by others to affect your free will. If you look at the list of wrongful uses of power (see Appendix 1), you'll see various avenues others can use to affect you, if the intent is there.

Throughout my journey, I've run into many examples in which people, including myself, were affected by others sending energy that was not appropriate. Depending on your sensitivity to energy, it might be obvious to you from the way your energy feels; or you could be oblivious to it, but find you're not happy, or maybe feeling depressed, or that nothing seems to be going right for you. My chosen role in sharing information about Wild Card Therapy has sometimes put me in a position of being the target of those, either in spirit or flesh, who don't want to see this information shared. I have removed curses and spells that were sent to me and to my family. Personally, I didn't notice a huge affect from them, but what's upsetting is that someone can send wrongful energy to anyone. Ignorance is not bliss in this case; a lack of acknowledgement doesn't lessen the affect. In fact, awareness and acknowledgement, in conjunction with the tools in this book, make you very powerful in protecting yourself from others who might try to impede your free will.

AT': Your free will might be to reject the existence of such things as curses, spells, hexes, and such, but they *do* exist regardless of your beliefs. They're based on the power of thought, and the more focused and intense the thought, the stronger the curse, or wrongful energy.

Personally, I don't believe in the trinkets, herbs, chants, and such which many people use to give shape and substance to spells and curses. Even so, having removed curses and spells from myself that were centuries old, I know they exist, and I know the trouble they cause. When they're created, regardless of the material objects used, their main power is a piece of awareness calved away from their creator, which gives them substance and longevity. In other words, the person who creates the spell, or curse, sends an ALP with it when they send it out into the world. Even if you don't believe in such things, it's still a good idea to reject any and all such thought energies which might be clinging to you, just to be on the safe side, especially since they follow you beyond the lifetime they were created in. They become more warped and potent with each lifetime, since the original ALP creates its own ALPs whenever it needs reinforcements.

For example, a friend of mine, who'd cursed her mate many lifetimes ago, was still being affected in this lifetime. In the lifetime when the curse was placed, she was in a male body and her mate, who is now male, was then female. In that lifetime, my friend's mate had left her, so she (who was then a he) cursed the mate to always return. Hundreds of lifetimes later they were still interacting, warped not only by the original curse, but by the many curses they'd laid on each other since. During this lifetime, my friend began to heal and wanted to break loose from her mate. Although she had grown both spiritually and mentally, and cleansed herself of all she could find to heal, this labyrinth of curses still bound them together, along with many generations of ALPs tending to the curses, and all the crud which had adhered to them. Releasing the original curse was just the beginning of the cleansing process, and it took weeks to clear everything away, including the atrophied pieces of herself which had been pinched off beneath them. Even so, she persevered until all this was finally gone, and she found herself whole and no longer clinging to a relationship which should have ended eons ago.

Removing Inappropriate Energy Ties or Energies

GM: Energy ties (see Appendix 6) are ties that bind us to someone who affects us. The only appropriate energy ties are those with our spirit mates that occur naturally and with no ill effects. Ties with others can affect us negatively, without our realizing it. To remove them, repeat the following: "I reject any energy or energy ties around me that are not appropriate, and call on Archangel Michael to deal with them appropriately."

AT': Energy ties cling to the outside of our shields, hindering our ability to see our choices clearly. They warp our views of ourselves and everything else around us, sometimes causing us to see what the creator of these ties wishes us to see instead of the truth. If you recite the above rejection and still feel things clinging or warping you, get angry and say: "Archangel Michael, deal appropriately with all wrongful attachments and those who have created them. I reject all attachments from outsiders because they warp my true pathway, and the pathway of those who have created them. If I am the one who created these attachments, I now release them and ask the forgiveness of those who were attached to me, requesting that you now clear them away, so the other and I can follow our true pathways unhindered by outside attachments."

Be firm in your desire to be cleansed of such attachments. Don't take no for an answer, since only your spirit mate and the True Creator have the right to be attached to you, and their attachments are internal, not external. Remember, it's impossible for us to find our true pathways when intruders, attachments, and ALPs unbalance us. If after doing this you still feel attachments to another, you may have pieces of yourself clinging to them or they to you. Ask Archangel Michael if such is the case, and if so, then use the release in the section below, "Reclaiming Lost Pieces of Self."

Removal of Psychic Parasites

GM: Psychic parasites can cling to our shields and our energy, affecting our ability to cleanse. To cleanse parasites, command your personal shields to create energy bubbles with the types of energy the parasites find most tasty, so they transfer their feeding from you into the bubbles, and then call upon Archangel Michael to deal with them appropriately. Once they are removed, call upon your Core Self to fill in all areas weakened by the parasites.

Strengthening Your Shields

GM: Having and keeping strong shields is extremely important. Upon completion of the above process, and regularly, you must strengthen your shields. Listed below are the steps for this.

1. Ask your Core Self to help with this and see pure light ignite in your centermost particle and begin growing outward, pushing out all that is not you and all you have outgrown.
2. Your Core Self will automatically fill in the emptied areas with appropriate energies and stop your shields' growth in their appropriate places.
3. Call on Archangel Michael and the Holy Spirit to sort and deal appropriately with all you've pushed out.
4. The only energies that should be flowing into you are from your core. Ask your Core Self and symbionts to rebalance you appropriately.
5. Repeat as necessary for strong shields, and trust your shields to know which energies to accept, or reject, for your highest good.

AT': If you're unsure of where your outermost particle is, don't be concerned, since your Core Self knows. Your Core Self automatically controls the rebirthing process; all you need to do is command that it be done. You can also modify your shields' energy resonance by simply commanding that it reject, sour, or block that which causes you harm emotionally or otherwise. If you trust your shields and yet feel something is getting through that shouldn't be, repeat the above steps focusing on the energy you want to stop, asking that as soon as that energy touches your shields it be transmuted with unconditional love, and rebounded back to the sender to begin the cleansing process. This refining process can be done as often as you feel the need.

Part II: In-Depth Cleansing

GM: Deep cleansing may not seem as straightforward as basic cleansing. If you find yourself getting upset or confused, take a few moments to focus by taking three slow, deep, cleansing breathes. Then, trust that your understanding of the process is appropriate. Remember that when using these techniques, you are never alone and you will receive support and messages from the other side to guide you to do what is appropriate. Trusting yourself is the key. No one's going to tell you you're wrong.

AT': If you feel you can't trust yourself in this process, think you're getting deceptive answers, use the steps in Chapter 8 to deal with deceivers and find a method for getting answers you can trust, but don't give up. By using the exercises in this book, you can remove hindrances to the truth, and learn to trust yourself again. For example, we've been working with a woman who was near her wit's end in trying to find peace and truth. There were many things hindering her from reaching the truth of herself, some of which were from outside sources and some from within, but after long, hard work she is finding herself once more. As she grows closer to being clean and whole, she's growing stronger and more loving in her relationships, and finding love for herself once more. So don't give up. Keep fighting for your right to be whole and clean and filled with self-love.

Balancing Paradox Directional Selves (PDSs)

AT': When dealing with PDSs that are hindering you, follow the steps below.

1. Wrap all problematic PDSs (see Appendix 4) in pure light quicksilver. This is the most pure and powerful form of light in existence and beyond, coming straight from the True Creator, and available to us on request.
2. Call on the Holy Spirit and the ivy of Saint Peter's gate to gather in the PDSs.
3. Visually, create a box from the pure light quicksilver, and line it with thick velvet to protect them from harm.
4. Visualize placing the PDSs in the box, and set it just outside your inner core, where outsiders can't harm it. They will still be able to whisper thoughts that are appropriate, but inappropriate thoughts won't be able to escape from the box.
5. There may come a time in your cleansing when your PDSs need updated information. When this occurs, ask Archangel Michael to

create a receiving sensor for them in their boxes so they can have an inflow of true and appropriate information to help you help yourself.

Deep Cleansing Between Layers of the Self

GM: When cleaning between your layers, it's important to clean between, in, and around all fifteen plus one layers. We have both inner and base sets of layers that require cleansing (see Appendix 3). Here is my personal approach to this type of deep cleansing.

1.   When I cleanse between, in, and around my layers, I visualize myself sitting in my high spot. Once there, I visualize a trap door into myself, and a chair I can climb into. I visualize myself seated in the chair lowering into a tunnel. This tunnel represents my first layer.

2.   In the tunnel, I visualize myself pushing through it with a rush of pure light in front of me filling all areas in and around the layer, enveloping everything in its way so it can be recycled as appropriate.

3.   Upon completion of my first layer, I sit in my chair, and lower myself to the next layer. Continue this process for all fifteen plus one inner and base layers.

4.   Upon completion, double check by simply filling yourself with pure light quicksilver.

My tunnels are circular, so I could exit the other end of my tunnel and be back at my chair. If I found anything stubborn, and the pure light wasn't able to push it out, I'd wrap it in pure light and call on Archangel Michael to deal with it appropriately.

AT': There will come a point in your cleansing when you find the division between layers and other parts of self a hindrance. When this occurs, call on the pure light quicksilver to ignite in and around all division points and shatter these barriers, asking Archangel Michael and the Holy Spirit to gather in any ALPs, other beings, or things which were hiding there, to ensure you are alone within yourself. A more in-depth instruction for this process can be found in Chapter 8.

Reclaiming Lost Pieces of Self

AT': Lost pieces of self are those parts we've given away to others through intense emotions, or pieces which have been suppressed internally by curses, spells, ALPs, or other things which have prevented them from interacting with your whole as they should. Although giving away pieces of self seems to be a natural occurrence, it can cause trouble because we're no longer whole. Some people call this "soul retrieval," but I avoid this term because it implies we've lost our soul, which is not possible. These pieces are not the ALPs previously spoken of, although ALPs can be found with them.

An example of lost pieces is when you fall in love so intensely you hate being apart. If the relationship ends, you may have trouble letting the other person go and wonder why, even after years, you don't seem to be able to get them off your mind. This is because part of you is still with them, or it could be that a piece of them is buried within you. Whatever the reason, these pieces need to be reclaimed for you to be whole; if part of them is within you, then you need to return that piece to them to become clean. Below are the steps to set things right.

The Dominion Angel Neraphasea (Nera is a nickname she accepts which no other angel answers to) is in charge of knowing what is you and what is not. She knows where each stray piece of you is, and can also tell the difference between you and your ALPs (although when dealing with ALPs she calls on the Holy Spirit, since her jobs is the individual, not their children). Unfortunately, she can't automatically gather in all the stray pieces of you, but can only seek specific pieces whose absence you are aware of. Neraphasea can, when directed, help you reclaim these pieces from any lifetime, including from past time rounds. If you don't believe in the time rounds, or in reincarnation, ask her to focus on specific types of events, such as those formed by romantic involvements, the birthing of children, or other instances. While this may not gather all your lost pieces, it will at least give her a sense of your desire to become whole again.

Note that you can't reclaim all lost pieces of yourself at once, in part because they're scattered, but also because the knowledge and memories they may return to you could be overwhelming if you reclaim

g. Allow yourself to reabsorb the memories or energies ∟ch these reclaimed pieces hold. This may take time, and you may have to shift your worldviews before they can be fully reclaimed.

Repeat these steps whenever you feel the need to reclaim or remove such pieces.

Chapter 3:
Relationships, Love, and Family

GM: Now that you believe your cleansing is complete, you are dealing only with your own energy; anything you feel is only you, with nothing clinging, or overlapping. Now you're ready to deal with your own baggage. Love, romance, and family are issues for everyone in one way or another. When we are growing up, we're taught to listen to our elders, to do for others so they'll like, respect, and love us. Loving ourselves is the key to health, happiness, and healing related to the issues in this chapter. If you have thought, said, or heard any of the following, this chapter can help you.

A thought can lead to emotions or feelings related to that thought. The following are some examples.

The Thought	**Emotions related to that Thought**
Don't act like that. What will people think?	- lack of control - need to be on guard - resentment
Thinking of your own happiness is selfish.	- guilt
He/she knows that hurts me.	- betrayal - anger - hurt - confusion
I can't believe he/she/they would do that to me!	- betrayal - anger - hurt - treated with a lack of respect

I can't be myself because they don't understand me.	- guilt - hurt - anger - not worthy of being who I really am - judged
My mom/dad/sibling/friend doesn't like it when I do that, and I want them to like me.	- unloved or unlovable - obedient - anger - hurt
I thought they were my friends. How could they do that?	- betrayed - angry - hurt
Nobody loves me.	- sad - lonely - unlovable - self-critical
I'm lonely.	- sad - hurt - lost

This list is by no means exhaustive, but it indicates how we often feel in relation to others. Look at the list, and you'll see a pattern of how others make us feel. In all the above examples, we blame others for making us feel the emotions related to the actions or statements. The key to loving yourself, and to having healthy relationships, is to take responsibility for your feelings. Understand that taking responsibility means not allowing anyone to make you feel anything unless you allow it. This seems like a huge responsibility, but once you get that mindset, your life becomes less complicated and actually easier emotionally, ultimately leading to happiness. You control how you feel, so you now hold the power that you were previously giving to others.

AT': In learning to take responsibility for yourself and your actions, try acting instead of reacting to situations around you. Choices open up in your mind's eye that you may previously have been blind to, fearing consequences others presented, instead of the outcome you hoped for. It's a good thing, caring about others, but you can't control how people think and how they react to you. All you can do is control your own actions, and in following your heart you may find yourself receiving the love and respect from others that you were missing before. Even if you don't receive it from others, you will love and respect yourself, because ultimately, it is we who judge ourselves during our life review once we are back in the light.

What Does it Mean to Love Yourself?

GM: I regularly come across people who when asked if they love themselves quickly reply *Yes*, but when asked what they don't like about themselves they answer just as quickly. This is a sign that they're not really showing love to themselves. Each time we think or verbalize statements related to what is "not good" about us, we are not showing ourselves self-love or unconditional love. Have you ever said or thought the following?

Thought	Effect of Thought
I'm too fat.	- rejecting who you are - disrespecting yourself
I don't like my hair.	- rejecting who you are - disrespecting yourself - creating situation where your soul needs protection, sometimes leading to weight gain which represents such protection

I don't like going there because
I can't do what they do.
	- limiting yourself
	- worrying about what others feel
	  rather than trusting yourself to
	  learn if you choose to

I'm not good enough.	- hiding from self - fear - disrespecting yourself

Every time you notice something about yourself that isn't up to the standard you feel it should be, ask yourself this question: "Am I doing the best I can within my control?" Focus on this question. When I say the best you can, I mean at that time of your decision or thought. If, right now, you feel you're doing your best at (for instance) eating healthy, getting exercise, and dealing with your issues (weight is one way the body and soul protect themselves), then you are.

If you answer yes to that question, then forgive yourself for not trusting yourself, and the process of your life. This will initiate the habit of showing love to yourself and giving yourself unconditional love. If you answer no, then why aren't you doing your best within your control? Are you purposely eating to get fat? It's unlikely that you're doing it for that reason, but there is a reason you're feeling the need to do whatever it is you're doing. In most cases, there are issues, or baggage, interfering with your feelings related to your size.

Whenever you feel negative emotions, i.e. emotions that interfere in a negative way like guilt, anger, betrayal, sadness, hurt, confusion, or hate, to name a few, you create negative energy in your body that can eventually develop into illness, pain, or disease. We have worked doing cleansing and emotional releases with many people who've healed their aches and pains, some of which have been hindering them for years. This was accomplished by identifying the location of the pain, and releasing the negative energy. If you're unsure what issue is affecting you, pinpointing the area of the body where the pain or disease is will help identify the issue. Louise Hay has a wonderful book called *You Can Heal Your Life*, which contains an extensive list of the emotional causes of illness, pain, and disease. Appendix 8 features a short list of some of the emotional roots to physical illnesses as given to us by Archangels Raphael and Michael

Once you embrace self-love, you'll find that relationships of every kind will change. People can sense how you feel about yourself, and will treat you accordingly. Recognize that we often project on others the way we feel about ourselves. Understand that those who judge you, hurt your feelings, or make you question yourself, are actually identifying and judging things they see in themselves, but they find it easier to judge others than deal with what they're unhappy about in themselves. They're not taking responsibility for their own emotions and feelings. Your understanding will allow you to feel empathy for them, rather than hurt, anger, or other negative emotions.

Now that you have more information about why others treat you as they do, and appreciate the importance of showing love to yourself, you'll find that negative situations will diffuse because you'll start acting for yourself, and not reacting to others. We can only control ourselves and our actions, not others, so by taking responsibility for ourselves, we choose whether and how we'd like to pursue our personal growth.

Having healthy relationships requires understanding that our emotions have a great affect on us. For example, when you meet with that friend with whom you are angry, your friend can sense that anger, and automatically puts up walls to protect himself from it. Usually those shields won't keep him from lashing out when he feels your anger, and starts to feel his own anger caused by guilt, or feeling that his actions were justified. Does any of this resolve the issue? No, it makes things worse. The only way to resolve the issue is for you to take responsibility for yourself, and release the associated negative energy (see section below on Emotional Release). Once it's released, you can look at the situation without these negative emotions cluttering things up. You'll begin to understand why he acted or said what he did. His statements or actions will not affect how you feel about yourself, and you will be true to yourself. A situation changes once you take responsibility for yourself, even if the other person's behavior remains the same; you have changed, which means the situation has changed.

Emotional Release

GM: An emotional release cleanses your body of the negative energy created by negative emotions. Depending on the issue that established the negative energy, deposits of this energy reside in specific areas of the body, creating weakness and increased possibilities of illness, or disease. Illness or disease is your soul's way of sending a message to the conscious mind that you need to do something. In most cases, it's related to loving yourself, and being good to yourself.

The release process below is a safe, easy way to deal with emotions, without having to relive the situation. All that is required is recognizing the feelings evoked at the time of the issue you're releasing. Emotions are held in what we call "emotions eyeglasses," a pseudo-Wild Card that holds emotions created for each situation or issue. Rather than having to consciously identify the emotions, know that they're held in your emotions eyeglasses and you don't need to be bogged down by them to deal with them.

AT': Pseudo-Wild Cards are spirit objects buried deeply in an individual, surfacing only when the person reaches the point on their true pathway so the pseudo-Wild Card can be wielded appropriately. They, like the other Wild Cards, are born of the True Creator's unconditional love for us, and cannot be used wrongfully.

Steps in Emotional Healing Release

GM: All humans, including you, act based on past experience and upbringing, so the decisions we make are based on those, whether they're right or wrong. When you are looking to forgive, remember that the person you're forgiving, even if it's yourself, was doing the best he or she could do based on his or her experience at that time.

Also remember that we can't do any better than our best, and as long as we're doing everything within our control to deal with an issue, we're doing the best we can do. *No one* can do any better than their best. Before moving forward with the steps, ensure your ALP mirrors are in place.

1. To get the most benefit from this release, you must be able to give forgiveness or ask forgiveness of those causing you to feel those emotions. Forgiving those who evoked the particular emotion(s) in no way condones their actions. Forgiveness of others is a show of love for yourself, and it also allows you to actively take back your power to choose whether or not you want to feel those emotions.

2. Once you have forgiven others, it's time to show true love to yourself by forgiving yourself for allowing them to make you feel those emotions. Realize that no one can make us feel anything unless we allow it. Also forgive yourself for not trusting yourself and your life process.

3. Once forgiveness is complete, ask your angel to take the negative energy associated with those emotions to the light for purification; you don't want to waste any more energy on them.

4. When you have completed the above steps, ask your angel to fill in the areas vacated with pure light quicksilver and ask the Holy Spirit to deal with all karmic remnants appropriately.

If you find that forgiveness of another, or even yourself, is difficult, call on the Debit Package Wild Card, place it between you and the other person or those parts of you not wanting to forgive, and ask it to activate and do all appropriate. The Debit Package will absorb the energy you're feeling from the other person or part of yourself and transmute it into unconditional love, making it easier to forgive.

When it's difficult to release intense emotions for various reasons, including continued behavior by those causing the emotion, call on Aunts Lawgivers and Keepers to do all appropriate.

AT': In trying to help people, many times I've come upon those who refuse to forgive people who hurt them, either because the wound is still too raw or because the person is still causing harm. I understand this reaction, but it hinders cleansing of the wound so it can begin to heal. In the case of someone who's still doing wrong, try to work with the authorities (police or others) to end their bad behavior to protect others from them. If the authorities can do nothing, call on Aunts Lawgivers and Keepers to deal with them in all ways appropriate. In cases where the perpetrator no longer does such things, or they have already left this earth and returned to the spirit side of life, know they have had no choice but to deal with their bad behavior (seeing what they did from their victim's viewpoint). In these cases, they can't fully heal until you find a way to forgive them. In either case, if you have trouble forgiving, it might be helpful to see what about their past caused them to be that way. Perhaps they themselves were abused as children, or spirits that caused them to see the world in a warped manner overlapped them, or there might have been karmic ties that removed all other choices. Whatever the reason for their actions, *you* can't heal until you learn to forgive.

GM: Once you have completed this release, you should feel lighter and have a better understanding of others' actions, or feel empathy for the behavior. This release allows you to take back your power, re-establishing responsibility for your own feelings, and no longer allowing others to cause you to feel anything you don't want to. This is also the start of understanding the importance of loving one's self.

Healing is done in layers; you heal what's at the surface allowing more to surface. As they present themselves, acknowledge your feelings and do the above release.

The Importance of Emotions

AT': Emotions are very important to your wellbeing, but when you let your emotions control you, instead of you controlling them, it causes trouble. In the years since I began to explore the techniques in this book, I've evolved to the point where my emotions are balanced, and patience is my most common trait. I have delved deeply into my mind and my past, healing the wounds which once caused me to react instead of act. Even so, there comes a point when intense emotions still surface. They are necessary to focus thought and project intent into the world or spirit realms.

At this point in my journey, I'm reaching for those intense emotions, and finding it hard to access them because my first tendency is to be patient and see things from everyone's perspective. This brings home the point that some people suppress emotions, rather than dealing with them. Even though I gained control of my emotions through patient exploration, and didn't suppress them, it's become difficult to call them forth and wield them when I have need. Emotions should be looked at, embraced as tools, and used to help you focus your thoughts.

The best way to deal with emotions is to understand them, and use them to do good. Just because an emotion is negative doesn't mean it can only be used to do bad things. For example, when you get angry because of someone else's actions, you don't have to strike out at them or blame them for something they might have done out of ignorance. Try using that emotion to tell the person directly how their actions made you feel, and ask them why they did it. Perhaps they didn't realize the consequences of their actions. In this way, when you're in control of negative emotions instead of them controlling you, they can do good things. If that doesn't work, you can use that anger righteously by calling on Archangel Michael, and others in the light, to clear the way for that person to see and understand his or her wrongful actions, and pray that his or her mind can be opened to find new and better approaches in the future. There is also a legion of angels called Aunts Lawgivers and Keepers (all aunts, not just me) who come together to bring justice and truth where it's needed. By calling on them and asking them to do all appropriate, amazing things can occur, but don't try to tell them what's appropriate. Leave it to them since they see things from a larger perspective than you do.

GM: I've called on Aunts Lawgivers and Keepers to do all appropriate in various situations, and each time I've called on them, I've had the fairest and most appropriate results. Whether or not you know if the situation is one they can deal with, simply asking them to do all appropriate will allow them to.

Cleaning House, Work Place, Telephone Lines, Objects

AT': I'm not talking about picking up a mop and scrubbing your floors, but rather making sure that no spirits, wrongful energies, emotional residue, or other such things are interfering with you and those around you. I'm not necessarily talking about haunted houses, but that is the extreme form of what I mean. Problems, such as a build up of old body energy left from intense emotions, or a lost soul drawn in by someone's ability to sense them (like a light in the darkness for them), can hinder the free flow of interaction between people in your house, your workplace, over telephone lines, as well as clinging to objects like your computer.

Let's talk about body energy residue first. A perfect example of residual body energy occurs when there are teenagers in the house. Have you ever smelled the bedroom of a teenage boy? The testosterone is overpowering. This is similar to what happens when the teenager overreacts and you end up arguing. Those emotions permeate the house remaining even after the argument is over, building up layer after layer. Any intense emotional confrontation, whether between parent and child, spouses, coworkers, or even if it's one-sided, causes emotional residue that remains until you send a pure light vacuum tunnel through the house to remove it. I recommend this be done weekly when there are teenagers in the house, or whenever tensions feel high. Another easy way to do this is to ask Archangel Raphael to use his pure light vacuum to cleanse your home.

Things with awareness, such as lost souls, psychic parasites, and other beings not bound materially, can be found in many places and objects, either hiding or having been drawn by the spiritual awareness of the people near them. There's no need to be afraid of such things; they are easily dealt with. As you reside in the material, it is your right not to have these beings around you uninvited. Wrap them in pure light quicksilver and call on Archangel Michael to gather them in, dealing with them appropriately by cleansing them and taking them to the light, or use the appropriate commands listed elsewhere for the individual being or object. Other things that might be involved are warped time (see Appendix 11), and portals to other realms that must be dealt with separately. With warped time, there may be spirits who wandered in and became trapped, unable to free themselves. Ask Archangel Michael to deal with all trapped, calling on their loved ones who are in the light to come speak with them, and ask the Holy Spirit to clear away all within the warped time before shattering and vacuuming it up. Portals can be either a problem or a delight, depending on your point of view and where the other end of the portal opens. In one instance, I dealt with a woman who was glad of the portal because she enjoyed taking pictures of the orbs that filled her home as spirits came and went from the garden of light, but other people have been scared of them since their house was continually filled with spirits. To deal with portals, ask Archangel Michael to create a gate across it and give you the key, that way you have a choice of having it open or closed. If you rent, make sure you leave the spiritual key behind when you move, so the angels can tend to the gate.

Elementals are a different issue, since their environment naturally overlaps ours, and they can be very beneficial. These beings exist in a state that is neither material nor spirit, but somewhere in between, present everywhere on the planet taking care of the Earth. Introduce yourself to the Elementals who live and work in your area. Use the same method you would when speaking with your Spirit Guides, but listen for their voices on the left side of your head, instead of the right. Get to know them and ask for their help in keeping your home or workplace clear of other non-material beings. Ask the Elementals about the power lines (ley lines, Earth's life force) which run through the places you live or work, and request that they realign these energy flows so they are beneficial to you, those around you, and the plants and animals you share your space with. When ley lines cross beneath a building, they can cause a column of energy to rise up into the air, cutting through the home or building. Although this is natural and necessary for the planet's health, it can cause trouble inside the home, so ask the Elementals and Archangel Michael to build a channel to shift the energies outside before allowing them to surface.

I also think it's a good idea to focus on the Internet, the chat rooms you enter, and what comes through your telephone lines. Many chat rooms, especially those dealing with spiritual subjects, are like magnets for lost souls and even people in the material who send wrongful energies. Since there is a wide variety of things which can come through your telephone line, set up a pure light quicksilver filter where your line leaves the main line and heads towards your house. If you've already visited such websites, I suggest calling on a pure light quicksilver vacuum tunnel to clean your telephone line, your computer, and your house. You may also want to do the cleansings found in Chapter 2 to rid your home or workplace of beings, objects, and energies which might have come through. Here too, once you have the filter in place on the phone line, ask Archangel Raphael to occasionally do a pure light vacuuming of your line, computer, home, and yourself to get rid of any energy build-up.

A good way to keep your home or workplace clean is to create a pure light quicksilver sphere of energy encompassing the entire property. You can also create these around yourself, and each member of your family (with their permission), as well as around your vehicles. The steps for this process are given below. I recommend you nurture your shields weekly in the beginning, and monthly thereafter to keep them strong. Re-birthing your shields annually is probably a good idea if you have teenagers in the house. Note that if something is appropriate to the needs of your growth, or the growth of those with whom you share the space, the sphere won't affect this. If you create these spheres around every member of your family, you can prevent things from clinging to them, and being carried into the sphere. When you have visitors, ask the sphere to bind whatever overlaps them, until that individual gives permission for a cleansing; otherwise, there's the risk of these things jumping off the one they rode in on and attaching to someone or something else in your home.

Follow these steps to create a protective pure light quicksilver sphere.

1. Call on the pure light quicksilver to ignite in the centermost particle of that around which you wish to create the shield.

2. Ask the pure light quicksilver to grow outward, pushing out anything that isn't appropriate (beings, energies, or objects) as it grows.

3. Picture the pure light quicksilver sphere growing until it covers every inch of the person or property you wish to protect. Visualize the sphere growing even beyond the boundaries, up into the air and down into the ground as well.

4. Call on Archangel Michael and the Holy Spirit to deal with anything and everyone pushed out by the sphere, then send a pure light quicksilver vacuum to clean up any residual energy, or anything else needing recycled.

Chapter 4:
Success

GM: Before you read this chapter, I'd like to share a story. Initially, we titled this chapter "Finance, Money, Career, Success." As soon as I sat down to begin writing, my left arm and hand started to ache and my stomach became nervous. I typed the chapter title, but couldn't go any further so I gave up. I couldn't write anything; my mind was blank. I thought for a minute and spoke with Aunt T'. Between us, we realized the problem was the title itself. Everything we had listed comes automatically with the type of success discussed in this chapter. I took the opportunity to use the Wild Cards and clear the way for its completion.

In learning about personal success, it's important that we are aware of factors throughout our lives that have affected us and our worldviews. Recognizing and understanding those factors allows us to do a review and inventory for ourselves, deciding what is acceptable to us and what isn't. Acknowledging the following as factors that can impact our worldview allows us to dismiss worldviews that are no longer relevant to us.

Beginning in childhood we are bombarded by systems established to teach us to ignore our own power and do as we're told. As children, our parents pass on to us their understanding of life and religion. This begins at birth, continues through our early development and is further entrenched by the school system. When we graduate from school, businesses decide whether we are employable based on whether or not we are a good risk to make them money. Companies say they want people who can work independently, but that independence stretches only as far as their policies allow.

Influences on the True Self and Worldviews: Parental Influence

GM: Our learning or programming, starts when we're very young, attempting to ensure that we "go with the flow" rather than use our own feelings and sense of personal responsibility to live our lives. We're told what to do, how to do it, and in many cases, if we don't do as we're told, we're punished by a time out, grounding, and even a spanking.

Parents play an extremely important role in their children's lives. Teaching them to make their own decisions, and learning from the consequences of their choices, is invaluable in helping them learn to use and trust their own feelings. Having said that, there are possibly dangerous situations from which children need to be removed to keep them safe. A situation like that is a time for speaking with children, helping them understand the dangers of the situation they were removed from.

As parents, we need to be in touch with our own feelings to ensure we're not transferring them to our children. Teaching fear to children, rather than helping them find their own power, is a dangerous precedent. To fear those in authority is the beginning of the "go with the flow" syndrome, and promotes the idea that it's acceptable for others to have power over us, to control us, and that our true feelings are worthless.

Judging our children is another trap. We need to allow our children to be who they truly are, and not expect them to be who we want them to be. Similarly, we need to stop judging ourselves and allow ourselves to be who we truly are. Judgment of self and others creates and further promotes the whole hierarchal structure that sustains adversity in the world.

School System Influence

GM: As we grow, and enter the school system, formal societal programming begins. We are introduced to another hierarchal system. We are graded as A, B, C, D or F/R students. Where I live, anything below a B is unacceptable; these students are labeled as requiring increased attention, usually from the parents rather than the school.

If we don't do well in school, or haven't embraced school as we're expected to, are we really failures? Could it be that we didn't totally accept the schooling system as it was, but recognized the need for change and worked towards being a catalyst for change as best we could? Is it possible we were actually following and listening to our true self, rather than blindly accepting the status quo?

Much of our family time is spent helping children with their homework. Our children have limited time during the school week to be children. The so-called improved curriculum and testing creates stress on our children and on family time. The purpose of the new curriculum is to increase our children's knowledge so they'll be better prepared for the business world. However, to be productive, happy adults, children must have the opportunity to be children, to learn from their surroundings and experiences. We all have common sense, and it's in childhood that we're able to get in touch with it. The nature of the school system and its teaching methods hinder our children from tapping into their own common sense.

Our school system is focused solely on the business world, funded by a government that seems to be in the back pocket of the business world. Business focuses on the material; the more profits you make, the better you are, the more powerful you are. That attitude makes people feel they are failures if they aren't materially successful. The hierarchal nature of business and government has created a society in which few have material wealth and many are the working poor. The working poor can't afford those material things the wealthy have; the hierarchy would come crashing down if they did. Those who aren't wealthy are kept in that position by those in power, challenged to meet their most basic needs. When you must put all your energy into meeting your basic needs, there is little energy left to challenge the hierarchy, or find your true self and voice.

The way we're treated as children, and raised, has a lasting affect on us. Through laws and societal pressure, our children are forced to endure the programming of not trusting their own feelings, but instead to feel what they're told to feel and do as they're told to do. Children aren't stupid, but our system isn't open-minded enough to think outside the box to teach children to be themselves. Having said that, in a hierarchal system, there is no desire to encourage children to learn in the way that best suits them, allowing them a position of comfort, making them less controllable. Where I live, statistics show that the dropout rate with this new and supposedly improved education system is increasing. Children feel like they're not smart enough, and the frustration and pain of academic failure overwhelms them, making them feel empty and lost—ideal conditions for being controlled.

Religious Influences

GM: We all have a basic truth within us that we feel drawn to find. In many cases, religion helps fulfill that need. What we believe is our own choice since free will choice is a gift from the True Creator. Religious institutions have worked hard over the years to get people to believe what the church wants them to believe. Hence, we have factions of a religion fighting against other factions over little things. Many religions have sacraments and rites that followers are required to participate in to be fully accepted into the religion. Those who choose not to participate in these sacraments, rites, or rituals may be told that God will judge them and their place in heaven will not be guaranteed. If they do anything contrary to what the religion sees as acceptable behavior, they are sinners, whom only that religion's God can help. Remember, the True Creator has unconditional love for you, always and forever, and no one has the right to tell you otherwise.

In my research and personal soul searching for my own truth regarding God and life, I've always been fascinated that we are told that God loves us, that it's not right for us to judge others, yet there is an acceptance that judgment is appropriate from God. The acceptance that we deserve the pain we feel, or the treatment we receive because it's payback for behavior that God will judge, is merely a fear of taking responsibility for our own behavior or standing up for ourselves. It's always easier to blame then to take responsibility.

This attitude also affects our children. At an early age, we teach them what is acceptable to God if they want to go to heaven. Fear is placed in them for things that, in many cases, are normal childhood behaviors or thoughts. Fear leads to guilt. We begin to feel that we are terrible, that we make God unhappy. This adds to our feelings of worthlessness. This creates a tendency to not value our own thoughts or feelings, resulting in a feeling or need to allow someone else to decide for us.

AT': It is from such attitudes that extremists and terrorists come, because they believe they have to do something extreme when they're told others are going against God's will. In the United States people have shot doctors and others who work in abortion clinics "murdering God's children," and so they become what they are taught to hate. In other lands, there are suicide bombers who believe they will be welcomed into paradise if they give their lives to blow up the enemy. By taking away people's ability to think for themselves and access the truths within them, society sets itself up to be attacked by such people. Think for yourself. Feel the truth within. Know that everyone you see around you is also a child of the True Creator, loved unconditionally. There are better ways to deal with those who break the sacred laws of existence, such as calling upon Aunts Lawgivers and Keepers to do their jobs, rather than taking the law into your own hands, and perhaps causing harm to something the True Creator needs to occur to bring about other things further down the line.

Hierarchical System Influences

GM: As we grow up and become responsible citizens, we're controlled by our surroundings. We are also controlled by our emotions. At this time of spiritual awakening and change, issues and emotions surface that may be difficult to recognize. Rather than seeing them as issues, situations, or emotions to be healed, one of three scenarios can occur. First, sometimes people embrace the feeling that they're not good enough, that all they're feeling and doing is their own fault and that they deserve whatever they're feeling. Second, they may place blame on others for their situation and not take the responsibility themselves. The third scenario is that in which there's an understanding that all experiences happen for a reason, whether for personal/spiritual growth, or lessons to be learned.

AT': Something else I've noticed, is that often when upheaval occurs in our lives it is our soul's way of pushing us out of our comfort zone. It's hard to reach for the new and unknown when we're comfortable in the lives we have. Breaking out of our inertia can be painful, but it strips away the old and outgrown to make room for new things needed for our growth. Do not fear change. Change only hurts if we fight against it.

GM: Taking responsibility is very important in healing and personal/spiritual growth, but it's more important to understand why we did what we did, to learn from our experiences. The most critical aspect of growth and healing is to forgive ourselves. Be honest with yourself; recognize that whatever situation you're in, you did the best you could do in that situation with the knowledge and experiences you had at that time. Understanding and forgiving yourself, allowing unconditional love of self, is very empowering and leads to personal success.

Dealing with Worldviews that are no longer True for You

GM: The following technique will help you recognize and reject worldviews that are no longer appropriate to who you are, and strengthen the worldviews you currently hold. Before you begin, call your inner core and your subconscious mind to attention and state the reasons for needing to do this. The subconscious needs to understand what you're doing it to help your growth; reassure your subconscious mind of the safety and importance of the exercise.

1. Make a list of worldviews that have been created or developed within you from birth to the present.
2. Next, list the present and true worldviews or beliefs you have as an adult, and crosscheck it against your original list.
3. To reject worldviews that are no longer true for you, and reinforce your true worldview, ask the Holy Spirit to deal with those parts of you not in agreement with your new worldview.
4. Fill in all vacated areas with appropriate core energies. Repeat the above steps for each worldview.

AT': It isn't easy to change your worldview, or even modify it, without understanding the original. It's well worth the effort, but in doing so you may find that you have to do many of the cleansing exercises previously discussed in the book to make room for the change. Without the aid of your subconscious mind, you may find yourself flinching away from this section of the book, which only means that there is a need to focus on it. Have perseverance and encourage your subconscious to see how these changes will benefit your growth spiritually and materially. Another way to deal with this is to ask your subconscious to see how these worldviews interact with your First Dream template, asking if they are appropriate or not to your true pathway. If they aren't, ask your subconscious to help you dismantle them with the above steps.

What is Success?

GM: Have you ever thought about what makes someone successful? I'm sure different people will give you different answers. There is, however, a common denominator for all. Successful people never give up on themselves, and they never judge themselves negatively. In your pursuit of success, don't judge your success based on someone else's notion of what that is. Unless you've lived in their shoes, their success is not comparable to yours. We have chosen our own paths and lessons to learn. Some may choose to live with an abundance of money, others with love, others with prestige, others with material comfort. But none of these is necessarily a sign of true success.

No matter what path we have chosen, success doesn't come naturally. The key to success is how you feel about yourself; that's what translates into personal success. There's nothing wrong with being materially well off, provided you understand that material goods are only valuable here in the material world, and that money doesn't automatically make you happy. The news often reports people with money committing senseless crimes, buying extraordinarily high-priced items, looking for their money to fill that empty spot inside.

Successful athletes, whose lifespan in their chosen sport is short, may do very well financially in that time, but they are still not able to stop the aging process and continue in their profession past a certain age. In some cases, this is a natural and accepted evolution; in others, athletes get their self-esteem and love from the adoration of fans. What happens when they are no longer an athlete, but an ex-athlete? Where does that leave their self-esteem and love? Some turn to drugs or alcohol to fill the void. Another example is executives who work eighty-plus hours a week. They can't spend a lot of time with their families because of their jobs. They wake up one day and find their family has left or grown up and they've missed the time when cherished memories are generated.

One huge lesson for us all was the tragedy of September 11, 2001, when the World Trade Center in New York was destroyed. That event was tragic and hard to understand, but many of us also learned from it. On September 10, we were thinking of ourselves, and all the day-to-day things in our lives: meetings, bills, shopping, etc. Once the initial shock passed, people started thinking more about their loved ones, how precious they are, how precious life is, and what is really important in life. People's priorities changed. Suddenly, buying that new item wasn't as important, nor was working overtime to get a particular task done. Petty disagreements became ridiculous in the whole scheme of things.

This shift in priorities was a silver lining to that dark cloud. Those who lost loved ones were as much heroes as those who died, and I thank them daily for their sacrifice. Their courage and ultimate love for all of us allowed us a chance to learn our lesson about what's really important in life, what leads to true personal success.

Life is a journey, and it's within our own control what happens to us, and how we deal with it. Success is truly a life-long journey and you should rejoice in all the successes of your life, and understand that life's trials are also needed to give us perspective.

Steps for Personal Success

GM: Here are the steps to creating enduring personal success.
1.   Identify the areas where your worldviews or beliefs interfere with your personal success.
2.   Recognize and rejoice in all your successes, even the little ones.
3.   Understand that there are no failures or mistakes, only opportunities for learning.
4.   Acknowledge that you're doing the best you can within your control and that you can't ask for anything more. Understand that your best one day may differ from your best on another day.

5. Loving yourself, and sharing yourself with others, is the key to success, and everything else (material goods, money, prestige, etc.) will follow.

6. Follow your heart. Follow your passions. Do for you, not for others. Be true to yourself. (This doesn't mean ignoring the needs of others, but rather making sure you do no harm to yourself when helping them.)

7. Don't do anything simply for the money, because you won't find what you're looking for, or what your soul desires.

The Meaning of Life

AT': To me, true success is growing into who you were born to be, and doing joyfully that which you came into this life to learn. In other words, the meaning of life is to find your true job and do it joyfully so those around you will be uplifted and better able to find their own true jobs in life. How do you do that? It's both easy and hard. Start by looking at your life so far. What is it that stirs your greatest passion and joy?

For me, it was helping others, but I couldn't do this until I'd come a long way down the road to helping myself. I missed out on extended schooling because I flinched away from it. I found that what I needed to learn couldn't be taught by others; it was within me and out beyond the bounds of our material existence. I wandered through life, barely able to function due to the molestation and rape which I'd experienced in my youth. Time after time, I found myself in situations dealing with spirit or psychic powers. Finally, I went to a hypnotherapist for help, and she gave me the tools that helped me uncover my true self. What has been written in this book are not her tools, since they merely cleared my way to finding what was inside me. Walking my pathway, I work with the angels, beings of light, who have helped shape the tools and exercises which are in this book.

Inner Seeking Countdown

AT': This is the first of these modified tools. Where the hypnotherapist would count me down from ten to one, I count down from fifteen, plus one, involving all the base layers of the self that need to be engaged, or shut off, to flow towards the knowledge being sought:

1. Relaxing and breathing deeply, in a place where you won't be disturbed, begin the countdown and add a "seeking phrase," for example, "I seek what is blocking my pathway," between each number. Don't be concerned if the phrase changes slightly as you count down; the part of you that knows is trying to help you arrive in the place you need to be.

2. Repeat the countdown as many times as you need to, until you feel yourself relaxed fully.

3. If you see flashes of images or colors as you do this, ask Archangel Michael and the Holy Spirit to deal with any and everything hindering you from reaching your goals. If the images remain, focus on them. Ask your knowing self how they fit into what you are seeking.

4. Reject any preconceptions that might warp the answers you receive. Demand the truth, and the truth behind the truth of self, all else, and all others appropriate for you at this time.

5. Explore these visions for as long as you need to gain the knowledge you seek. Don't be concerned about becoming lost, since your conscious mind will awaken you when you're ready, without the need to count yourself back up.

AT': If you fall asleep during this process, don't be concerned, but do pay attention to any dreams or emotions you wake up with. Use them as clues in your seeking. Enjoy the process and don't become frustrated, since frustration is a hindrance.

Chapter 5:
Emotional and Physical Pain:
Death, Grief, and Fear

GM: This chapter is one everyone can relate to at one time or another in their life. We'd all like to avoid, rather than deal with, hurt and pain. While dealing with loss through death or illness is never easy, an understanding can help bring peace of mind and enable you to cope better with such losses.

Emotional and Physical Pain

GM: We've all experienced or witnessed emotional and physical pain at some time. Realize that physical pain usually has an emotional root, and emotional pain only hurts as long as you allow it to go unhealed. I've spoken with many in my journey who have had horrendous lives, much of which I couldn't imagine enduring. With everything they've experienced, they've reached something deep inside them that we all have, but might not be aware of. We all have an inner strength that once tapped into, makes everything possible.

There are no issues or struggles too great for us to conquer on our true pathway. Our struggles make us who we are. When you think of all you've been through, realize that you're still here, reading this book to help yourself live an even better life. That's something to be proud of, a sign of love to yourself. That's worth getting excited about, because once you've healed those emotions, then the road ahead is brighter. In fact, every time you heal an issue or incident, your road gets a little brighter. In reading this book, you're taking the initiative to heal. You've already tapped into your inner strength, perhaps without realizing it.

Shift your perspective to, "*Yes* I am strong," rather than focusing on, "I am weak, I have all these unhappy or scary things to confront." As long as you don't consciously give up on yourself, I guarantee your soul will never give up on you, nor will the True Creator. We have much support from the other side, including Guardian Angels whose goal is to see you happy and healthy. They will help guide you when you're feeling like you don't know which way to go or when you're feeling alone.

Meeting Your Guardian Angel

GM: Now that you have completed a cleansing of your energy, it's easier to communicate with your Guardian Angel. To connect, just follow the steps below. When communicating with your angel, remember that it might take a few times to open those communication channels, because the energy of Guardian Angels vibrates at a higher frequency then ours. Calling on the pure light quicksilver to ignite and clear the channel will also help. Communicating with angels requires us to raise our vibration, and the angel to lower theirs to meet at a point where the channel is clear.

1. Find a time when you're not going to be disturbed and get comfortable. Take three deep, slow, cleansing breaths. Breathe in through your nose and out through your mouth so deeply that your stomach moves. This will help clear your mind and relax you.

2. Say to yourself that you want to meet your Guardian Angel, and ask for his or her name.

3. Take the first name that pops into your head, regardless of whether it sounds familiar or odd. First thoughts are how many on the other side communicate with us. This is also an opportunity for you to trust yourself and your instinct.

4. Once you have a name, confirm by asking whether that is the name of your Guardian Angel. If you get a *Yes* through first thought, you can be assured it is your true Guardian Angel. Do the following two confirmations: i) Confirm that the name you received is your Guardian Angel. *Yes* or *No*? Ask this question eight times. If you hear *Yes* eight times, proceed to next confirmation. ii) Confirm that your Guardian Angel is working towards the True Creator's First Dream True United Destiny. *Yes* or *No*? Again, ask eight times. If you get *Yes* eight times with no hesitation then you can be assured you have connected with your true Guardian Angel and can begin conversing with him/her. You can ask for a message, or ask

them to show you unconditional love and feel the warmth, peace, and calm of their presence. *If* the answer is *No*, or you don't get a response, then chances are that you haven't connected with your angel. Focus on what you feel when you're communicating with the one supplying the name. If you feel fear or uneasiness, call on Archangel Michael to deal with whoever it is appropriately. Then repeat the above steps to try to connect with your angel again. Whether you connect with your angel or not is your choice, but know that they're always there for you, even if you're not aware of them.

AT': The above steps can also be used to connect with your spirit guides. It's important to learn how to trust yourself when hearing first thought, but if you haven't cleared away all that overlaps or clings to you, the answers you get may not be from guides or angels. Here are a few rules to follow when interacting with those beyond.

1. Angels and others in spirit speak to us through the area of our brain near the right ear.
2. Angels' names are not human names, except in cases such as Gabriel, Raphael, Michael, et. al. whose names have been incorporated into our world. If you ask for an angel's name and receive something like Paul or Margaret or Rufus, you may have connected with your spirit guide instead of your Guardian Angel. A spirit guide is also a good thing, but know the difference. Spirit guides have human souls, and their own pasts here on Earth, which influence the answers you may receive from them; their energies are different from angels'.
3. There are other spirits out beyond whose job it is to teach those of us here on Earth. They are neither Guardian Angels nor spirit guides, but come and go throughout our lives when we have need of them. If asked, they will identify themselves.
4. There are also messenger spirits who bring spirit items or messages to us. When spirit items are offered, they should be dealt with by asking your Core Self if it is appropriate to accept them at this time. If the answer is *Yes*, then ask Archangel Michael to cleanse them

first so their energy is clean and won't warp your own. Next, reach out to accept the item and bring it to your chest, absorbing it into your whole so that it helps you as it was intended to do, from within. Then ask your Core Self and symbionts to rebalance you appropriately with this new energy. If the answer is *No*, then call upon Archangel Michael to deal appropriately with the gift and the gift's messenger so they never again come near you.

These are the good spirits and souls you may hear from when seeking, along with a list of other voices you may hear within your mind (see Chapter 7 under "Sources of Thoughts"), but there are others who are not appropriate who may try to influence you if you haven't cleansed yourself of their attachments or energies. You may not always be able to discern these others by feel, so it's a good idea to keep asking for confirmation. True and honorable beings from beyond don't mind being asked for confirmation repeatedly, but the false ones become irritated and will try to guilt you into stopping. This is a sign that they are wrongfully attempting to influence you, so reject them and call upon Archangel Michael to deal with them appropriately.

Death and Grief

GM: About three weeks after completing this chapter, there was a death in my family that put my beliefs to the test. As well, I had the opportunity of speaking with other people to get their experiences, which I share later in this chapter.

Death and grief cause a lot of pain for people. One thing I find comforting is knowing that death is not truly an end, but a continuation of the spirit's journey. Having an understanding of where we go when we pass, or where our loved ones go, brings great comfort. Following up the earlier example of the tragedy of September 11, 2001, there was the appropriate number of angels to help guide everyone to the garden of light or the entrance of heaven. I remember when my Nanny (grandmother) was in the hospital after a stroke, and a few days from her passing, she'd talk and reach out to something. At that time, I didn't have the awareness or knowledge I have now, but I always knew it was my Uncle, who had predeceased her. I found great comfort knowing she would be taken care of when she left the earth plane and her ill body. The night following my Nanny's passing, I woke up in the middle of the night, and clearly saw my other Grandma standing in front of me. She didn't say a word, but I knew she was there to let me know that my Nanny who had just died was all right and that I shouldn't worry about her. That was my first encounter with seeing a spirit, and it was memorable because I found such comfort in it.

Another form of communication from loved ones on the other side is through dreams. Many find it a way to let their loved ones know they're doing well, without scaring them. If you find yourself having dreams that are hurtful or unhappy related to loved ones passed, question whether or not you have unfinished business with them. Many times our guilt, anger, fear or distress related to them, causes us to dream unhappy dreams. If this is the case, identify your feelings, and use the release in Chapter 2 to heal those emotions. You'll find your dreams will be much more pleasant. In many cases, those I've worked with in this regard have felt or smelled their loved one(s) around them.

When our loved ones go to the light, they reconcile their life with us. All issues from their life on earth are released, so they want you to release and heal from those issues too. They don't hold grudges, and don't want you to hold anything that might hinder you from walking your true pathway. Remember also that grieving is a natural process and the time for grieving is very individual, so give yourself the time you need to grieve. When you feel you've been grieving too long, look at the above for possible ways to help you heal.

When our loved ones pass, we can help ensure they go right to heaven, or to the light. A friend was telling me about an experience of hers, where her loved one, recently passed, came to her daughter, but hadn't gone to the light yet. When her daughter saw the loved one passed, she had sad feelings related to them. My friend had the loved one come to her (via a medium) feeling sad, guilty, and confused about their passing. Archangel Michael was called to help, and after educating the loved one, and with the support of Archangel Michael, she was able to assist her loved one into the light. The next day, her daughter said she could still see this loved one, but the feelings related to seeing her were happy, rather than sad. As well, this loved one came again to my friend (again, through a medium) where she was described as "glowing and peaceful." This was proof for her that her loved one was in the light, which brought great comfort.

The majority of people who pass on go directly to the light. In cases of tragic or unexpected death, there is a slight chance that they don't go directly to the light. It's important for spirits to go to the light where they can receive healing. Once healed, they are able to move and communicate much more easily than when clinging to the earth plane unhealed. You can help a loved one to the light by calling on loved ones already in the light, as well as Archangel Michael, to help them and by expressing the importance of their going to the light and returning after they're healed if they wish. The point of the preceding example was to let you know the process, so you realize the power you have in ensuring a loved one receives healing by going to the light.

In some cases, strong religious beliefs prevent people from going directly to the light, because many religions focus on God judging us when we pass on. If you've done things in life that you feel are going to disappoint, or that you're going someplace besides heaven, then you won't be in much of a hurry to get there. God does not judge us. Our contract with God is that we must take responsibility for ourselves. In taking responsibility for our behavior, we agree to learn the lessons we have chosen to learn, and will learn in this life or the next, hence there is no reason for judgment. As said in previous chapters, taking responsibility for our life means keeping the power God has provided us with to be happy and follow our pathways unhindered.

Projecting Your Spirit

GM: Once connected with your guide or angel, you might want to try projecting your spirit to heaven. This isn't astral traveling, because you're still in full control of your material body. I've tried this and it was amazing. In my experience, my guide and I were sitting beside a brook and I could feel my Nanny coming up behind me. That in itself was a wonderful experience, but it got even better. I thought that while we were in the area, we could stop by to see the True Creator. So that's what we did. Off we flew and within seconds I was in the presence of a huge energy. I could sense that I was being called to come closer by the True Creator, so I did. I could feel myself showered in His energy. At this point, I felt my time was going to be cut short by family commitments, so I thanked the True Creator and moved on. Next, we went to see Archangel Michael and Archangel Raphael, because I don't normally see them when working with them. Again, within seconds they both were standing in front of me, where we had a short conversation. Shortly, my sense proved correct, and my daughter came into the room where I was doing this. Throughout this adventure, I was fully aware of what was going on around me. In fact, I could hear my husband snoring beside me the whole time.

To try this yourself, follow the steps below.

1. Go to your high place identified in Chapter 2, or a place where you can feel comfortable and safe without being disturbed.
2. Identify where you want to go. Allow your intent and desire to guide you, without the limitations of earthly choices.
3. Call on your guide and all others appropriate to join you on your journey.
4. Visualize yourself flying. It's very individual, but I saw a light that I flew toward. Trust that you know where to go.
5. Heaven looks different to different people, so if you feel you're there, trust that you are. Take some time to enjoy the feeling of being there, and don't be surprised by who might come to visit or meet you. To get the most out of this experience, be open to what you're doing and trust that you're safe and protected. You are the only one who can limit your experience.
6. When you're ready to come back, just open your eyes and focus on the world around you.

Fear

GM: At one time or another in everyone's life, fear has controlled us, if only for a short time. Fear in itself isn't a bad thing; it keeps us aware and cautious when it's appropriate. But when fear controls our lives, there's a problem. As we've seen in previous chapters, things outside ourselves can create fear. Being overlapped by spirits who are lost or scared can make us feel their fear, as well as past life traumas. Unreleased ALPs can recreate the fear we felt when they were created if we encounter similar situations.

If you find you have unreasonable fear, fear that controls your life, this checklist may help you find its root.

1. Cleansing complete? Ensure that the fear is truly your own, and not something overlapping you. You can only affect that which is truly you.
2. Unreleased ALPs? Again, those kids aren't part of you anymore, but if they're clinging, they can still have an affect. The memories are yours, and if they surface, you can heal them by using the technique in Chapter 2.
3. Think back to the situation in which you first felt that fear. Have you released the negative energy around that situation, including releasing ALPs, healing those parts of self clinging to fear and needing reclaiming and all else that is hindering you from walking your true pathway?
4. Is the root of the fear related to a past life? If you can't find the root in this life, then a past life incident is likely the cause. In Chapter 8, we'll discuss an easy way to heal past life situations that are impeding your present life.

Remember that all the emotions identified in this chapter are natural and that we all feel them at one time or another. In themselves, they are appropriate; what's important is how we deal with them. We choose to allow them to control us, or to use the tools introduced in this book to take back control and responsibility for ourselves.

AT': No matter how fearful or painful healing can be, there is joy and growth waiting beyond. Persevere, grow into joy and don't allow the negative to turn you away from your chosen path.

Reclaiming Parts of Self

GM: I placed this section in this chapter, because many emotions ignite when once suppressed parts of self begin to surface. These can reveal themselves through a variety of bodily sensations, as your conscious mind tries to flinch away from these unknown parts. ALPs calve away quickly, enhancing the emotions and creating even more ALPs. There's nothing to fear about these parts of you being reclaimed, but few minds readily embrace the unknown when it arrives suddenly. People tend to cling to the known, which is why the body reacts with pain to force you to pay attention.

In most cases, you'll need a cleansing because of the new ALPs born when pieces of yourself flinch away from embracing and reclaiming parts of yourself, or because they have no wish to continue down this new pathway. Perhaps they fear what you will be capable of once you embrace these abilities. Either way, once they flinch away, these ALPs are no longer part of you. These stirring ALPs may reveal hidden memories, or overlapping, which could be what was suppressing these parts of yourself. In these cases, there may be karma to deal with, as well as the ALPs and outsiders.

When you ignore or flinch away from parts of yourself that are surfacing, your body may echo the same sorts of pains and discomforts you would feel if you needed a good cleansing. Do the cleansing spoken of in earlier chapters. If this doesn't relieve the symptoms, then the discomfort is more likely from the surfacing of abilities which you had no idea were yours.

Below, are the steps to reclaiming those parts of yourself that are calling for attention.

1. Call upon the pure light to ignite in and around all parts and particles of you that hinder you from reclaiming this part of yourself.
2. These parts are now ALPs and must be removed, so call on the Holy Spirit to take them. If he can't, then call on Archangel Michael and his legions to wield their weapons of pure light and slice between them and you, cutting them free. Ask Archangel Michael to push the ALPs out toward the Holy Spirit.
3. Once they've been removed, call on the pure light quicksilver to fill in all places emptied, and remove any barriers between you and this reclaimed part of yourself.
4. Now call on your Core Self, your appropriate symbionts, and mitochondria to embrace this reclaimed part of yourself and

rebalance you, burning clean appropriate channels so you can consciously access it.

5. Once you've rebalanced, ask your mitochondria and other symbionts to realign themselves and incorporate this new part of yourself. If you're still feeling anything odd, do a normal cleansing and then repeat the above steps.

AT': Some people call this soul retrieval, the reclaiming of parts of self, which is fine if they recognize all the variety of parts that need reclaiming. There are the pieces, which we send outward or attach to others (spoken of in Chapter 2), the suppressed parts that Gail Marie spoke of. For example, we worked with a woman whose suppressed pieces were surrounded by a cement structure, guarded by spirits who would only allow that part to be reclaimed when she proved she was ready. Once she has proven this by naming the piece of herself within the cement, the guardian will dissolve the cement, help her reclaim that part, then leave.

Reclaiming Inner Children, Teens and Adults

AT': Along with the suppressed pieces of self and those we send outward, there are also the parts of self that I call inners. Inner children are the best known, but there can also be inner teens or inner adults from this life or past ones. They are distinct from ALPs in that they are still part of us, and must be reclaimed for us to be whole. They are also distinct from suppressed parts of self in that they appear as whole beings, with their own emotions and reactions, but they aren't whole. They are stuck in the past, stuck at the point in time when they flinched away from us, and must be reclaimed before they can grow. For example, I was working with a woman who'd asked me to help her discover the reason she sabotaged relationships. She was with a good man, but was finding herself repeating the process of driving him away. During this process, we came upon an image of herself as a teenager which had more substance and emotion than an ALP, and she remembered the time in her life. After dealing with the forgiveness of the young man who had hurt her at that time, I had her talk to her inner teen and call her home (see steps below). We had to repeat this process several times with other inner teens, and even inner adults, from nearly every time she was traumatized in a relationship. A few weeks later, she told me how much things had changed, and how happy she and this man were together.

These inners must be dealt with in a slightly different manner than pieces and suppressed parts, because they are more fragile emotionally. After removing all the ALPs surrounding them, follow the steps below to reclaim them and begin their growth.

1. Once you have identified what you see as an inner, whether child, teen, or adult, talk to it. Tell it how you survived the incident that caused it to flinch away, and how much you have grown since. Tell it if you have forgiven those who caused you the original pain, and that you hope it forgives you for putting yourself (of that time) in such a situation. Tell it also that you love it dearly, and are not whole without it.

2. Once you have convinced it of the truth of these things, open your arms and call it forward. Embrace this inner and fill it with love as you absorb it back into you.

3. Ask Neraphasea and your Core Self and symbionts to help the inner merge into you appropriately, then rebalance your energies as the inner begins to grow into the person you are now.

4. Check for ALPs that might flinch away as you reclaim these inners, and do any of the other releases needed to clear the way for the inner to cease being an inner and become part of your whole.

Claiming Spiritual Power Objects

GM: The above is similar to claiming a spiritual power object that has been hiding deep within you awaiting the appropriate time to rise up for your use. For example, a friend of mine began feeling pain in her shoulders and neck. The cleansing routines did little to ease her symptoms. Finally, I asked if the pain was masking something appropriate that was rising to the surface, and got a *Yes*. When we looked closer, we found it was spiritual objects that had been waiting for her to evolve to the point where she could use them to help herself and others. Once we recognized this, we needed to clear away a few karmic ties around her inability to access these objects in the past, then clear away all ALPs flinching from using these objects. Soon, she was able to access them for the benefit of all. Using the method for reclaiming parts of yourself from the section on Reclaiming Parts of Self, replacing "parts" with "objects," you'll find the object can be accessed and the pain will fade.

AT': These spiritual objects are what I call pseudo-Wild Cards, individual tools born from the True Creator's energies for your needs. When you claim them, you need to understand what their abilities are in order to fully use them for self or for helping others. Not everyone seems to have these, but for those who do, they are invaluable to claiming your personal power and true jobs, so enjoy.

Chapter 6:
Karma, Past Lives, Cycles

AT': There is a common saying, "what goes around comes around," and that is a simple definition of karma. With karma, the way you treat others or act will come back to you threefold or more. So, if you're mean or rude, you can expect at some point in this life or the next to receive that treatment in return. It also works for positive forms of karma or behavior. For example, if you do good in your life, you'll receive good in this life or the next.

Having defined karma, it's important to understand that positive (credit) or negative (debit) karma can both hinder us from walking our true pathway. Debit karma can make our lives difficult, as things may not go according to schedule; it may seem that something's always going wrong, even with the most organized of plans. Similarly, credit karma can also hinder us from our true pathway, in that something is owed us that has yet to be repaid. That unpaid debit can interfere with our plans for life. An exaggerated example of this is typically played out on TV shows, in which someone saves another's life. The person whose life was saved feels he is indebted to the one who saved his life. Throughout the show, we see how disruptive it can be having someone paying back their debt. In this example, the indebted one is always under the feet of the other. He doesn't allow the "hero" to do anything for himself, thus leaving the "hero" powerless. The "hero" can't walk his true pathway because the indebted one is trying to do it for him, so he ceases to do and learn for himself.

Understanding that debit or credit karma can hinder us from walking our true pathway, we want to release and be clear of all karma. Below, you will see the steps for balancing your karmic scale. This method won't remove the karma from issues that need to be healed, or from lessons that still need to be learned, but it will clear the scale of karma.

The very nature of karmic credit means that there is an attachment to someone who owes the debt. To release karmic credit, you must believe that no one owes you anything for any of the good things you've done in this life, in any past life, or in the future, and that you reject any karmic debts that may be clinging to you. The truest reward for doing good things for others is the way it makes you feel, not how they react. Doing good things as a means of gaining recognition from others sets you up for a fall from your own soul rebelling against the karmic reverb generated. One way to avoid this trap is when you do something good and someone says they "owe you," tell them to either "pay it forward" to someone else in need, or say that it's your job as a human being and you've already been paid in full by your Creator.

It seems, however, there's still something about the money issue that eludes us. While clearing away karma helps in the spiritual sense and protects us from karmic payback, it seems to beat against a brick wall where society and money are concerned. Everywhere you look you see people seemingly being rewarded for doing bad things, when those who do good get beaten down. Remember that humanity and our societies evolved during the Angel Wars (which are now over), and so these may be traps and pitfalls that have not yet been rooted out and dealt with. This knowledge doesn't help those of us trying to do good and help others, but it lends a ray of hope that this too will heal as more of us become clean and whole. As our numbers grow in wholeness and light, we can only hope that society begins to evolve to reflect this as well.

For those of you wondering what the Angel Wars were, these five wars each happened when various factions of angels rebelled. The first war is well known since it's mentioned in the Bible, but its details and the story of those that followed are lesser known. These wars are now over and the majority of the rebels are once more in the light doing their true jobs, so I will leave the telling of that history to another book. This book is for cleansing and healing, not for dredging up the past, so be patient with me. Let's focus instead on the job of healing ourselves and humanity.

Steps for Clearing Your Karmic Scale

GM: Here are the steps to clearing your karmic scale.

1. Visualize your karmic scale. It varies for individuals. For me, it was an actual scale with blocks on either side. Someone I worked with saw a half circle, with two different colors on either side. Whatever you visualize is acceptable. If you can't visualize this, then believe that focusing on it will make it so. The more you believe in the reality of the next steps, the more power you'll add to the thoughts, and the more successful you'll be.

2. Trust yourself with whatever you visualize, and focus on the credit and debit karma. Credit karma usually seems light, or has less weight than debit karma. Remember that even good karma hinders your growth since it binds you to those who believe they owe you.

3. Once you have distinguished which is which, hold the Debit Package Wild Card, activate it, and place it on the debit side of the scale. Watch the karma dissolve until there's none left, or until the color on that side is white. Then take the Debit Package and place it on the credit side of the scale. Once again, watch it dissolve until there's nothing left, or the color is white. In my case, the scale itself dissolved.

4. Call on the Holy Spirit to clear away any and all karmic remnants, and ask Archangel Michael to clean anything between the karmic stuff and you.

5. Call on your inner core to fill in all areas vacated with appropriate core energies.

We carry karma to this life from past lives and into future lives if it isn't released by asking forgiveness of those it was created with, or by giving forgiveness to those who harmed us. Forgiving self is an important aspect of releasing karma once forgiveness has been given or received. If we aren't able to forgive ourselves for our role played in creating the karma, then we're clinging to it, accepting the karmic affect on us.

For example, if in a past life you killed someone, you have created a debit in your karma. To release this debit in your life, you must ask forgiveness from the person you killed in that life. Ask the person's soul for forgiveness, and take your first thought as the answer. Later in this chapter, we'll discuss a way of identifying past life issues, releasing their karma, and healing those emotions.

AT':   In karma, the responsibility for the harm lies with the one to whom the debit clings. If a merged spirit or any spirit overlapping you pushed you into doing something wrong, the debit is theirs, not yours. Of course, humanity's laws don't see it like that, so you'd have to pay the debt to society anyway, but those who record debit and credit on the scales of karma understand and assign it correctly.

Jesus Christ Credit Card

GM: This credit card will give you instant karmic credit for eternity and before. It not only reaches past credit and debit across eternity, but it also reads the desire within your intent to forgive and be forgiven. The power of this card is based on your conscious desire for forgiveness, from the point of receiving the credit card onward for life. There are two types of situations when this credit card is extremely appropriate for balancing karma (yin and yang).

First, it's appropriate for those who absolutely refuse to forgive someone else, or who have caused harm to another and are unable to forgive themselves. The credit card will activate the Debit Package Wild Card. When the Debit Package is activated, even though the person refuses to forgive, the person holding the card still has a chance to heal. For those who want to heal, or try to heal and are being hindered by others not wanting to forgive them, they can still heal regardless of the conscious lack of forgiveness of the other. For example, if I embezzled money from you and you hated me for doing it, you might find yourself unable to forgive me because of the hardship you endured as a result of my actions. My being open to Jesus Christ's credit card, plus my desire to heal and not harm others, gives me the opportunity to heal and get my life back on track.

Second, the card is appropriate when dealing with those who are transgressing and causing harm, but who don't want to stop and don't care if they receive forgiveness or not. The way the card works is, once received and the past karma is cleared away, the weight of that lifting allows for clearer thought and choices so that the need for healing can be seen by the individual. The card will activate the appropriate Wild Cards, so they'll receive credit from that moment backwards as soon as they accept the credit card from JC. The affect of the card is to clear the way for free thinking so that better choices might be seen from that nanosecond forward, and the card then judges their desire and conscious intent as to whether they continue to choose to harm others, or choose healing. At the moment of receiving Jesus Christ's credit card, your past debts are wiped clean, but when you deliberately harm someone in the future, it will not cover that karma until you truly seek forgiveness.

For example, if you harmed someone, and after having done it received one of JC's credit cards, it will clear the karma so you may see the harm you did and become regretful of your actions. If the person you harmed refuses to forgive you, and yet you seek to change your life, the credit card can clear the way for you to start healing.

AT': JC's credit card is for karmic and spiritual debts, but if you have broken humanity's laws then you must still pay your debts to society or to the ones you've harmed.

Getting Your Credit Card from JC

GM: Below are the steps to receiving your credit card.
1. Complete the appropriate cleansing and releasing commands.
2. Call upon the true Jesus Christ to come to you and ask him for one of his credit cards. Whether or not you see him, feel him or sense him, know that your thought intent is what makes it happen.
3. Accept the credit card from him, and hold it to your chest allowing all appropriate energies to be absorbed from the card.
4. When you are absorbing the energy, the following words are a message from Jesus Christ for us: "Now is the time to start asking for the forgiveness you always wanted and now to mean it, take it all and wrap it with my love."
5. Open up all appropriate parts of self to allow the card to do its job of clearing out all the karmic crud, and all else appropriate for it to deal with.
6. Once again, call all appropriate Wild Card therapy commands and releases. Then, fill in all areas vacated with appropriate core

energies. Call on your Core Self, mitochondria, and symbionts to rebalance your energy appropriately.

AT': The quote above was given to us by Christ himself, but to get a credit card you need not believe in Christ as Christians do, nor do you have to believe in karma. Christ is a real being, the Christed One, the High Commander of Spirits and Souls, and He believes in us, even if we don't believe in Christianity. As for karma, it boils down to forgiveness. If we don't forgive those who cause us harm, or ask forgiveness for the harm we cause others, we can never fully heal ourselves. It's that simple.

It must also be noted that when you ask for a credit card you may be offered more than one for various reasons. In one case in which Gail Marie was helping a woman receive a credit card, the woman didn't believe in karma, so Christ offered her three cards and allowed her to take the one she felt comfortable with. In another case in which I was helping someone get their card, she was offered two, one for herself and one for a being who was overlapping her, clinging near her heart chakra. Once this being accepted the card, Archangel Michael was able to cleanse and remove it without trouble.

Past Lives

GM: We have all lived past lives. In fact, we've lived many time rounds, fifteen to be exact, and we are in the plus-one time round now. Time rounds are most easily explained using an analogy to garlic. The garlic is made of individual cloves. Think of each time round as a clove of garlic, with many past lives in each clove.

There may be a few cases when new souls are born, but that's rare and even they have been born in other time rounds. Sometimes you might see someone on the street and think you know them, but you also know that you've never seen them before in this lifetime. Your soul is recognizing their soul. You likely knew them or interacted with them in a past life. Almost everyone we meet or see in this life we have encountered in past lives. My husband and I have been in thirty-three lives together, but not always married, and not always me female and him male. I have also been in forty-three lives with my oldest daughter and twenty-four with my youngest, but not always in the role of mother.

For the purposes of this book, the important thing to realize about past lives is that they affect our present life. Any feelings you have related to negative emotions described earlier in this book have likely been experienced in past lives and require healing. Until past life issues are healed, you will have those lingering emotions, whether you heal them in this lifetime or not. Remember, the only way the past can cause you harm is if you avoid it. Seeing it, acknowledging it, you can heal and then move on. For example, I was working with someone who had an artificial leg, and said he was having phantom pains from the amputated limb. We identified a past life in which his leg was blown off during a war. We were able to heal the issue from that past life, which eased the phantom pains, but I'm sure the pain will return because of other past lives in which that leg was also lost.

If you feel fear, or guilt, going through cycles of behavior and/or relationships, then chances are good that there are past-life issues that need to be healed to overcome those feelings.

Below are some methods for finding out about past-life issues requiring healing, without having to go through any kind of regression or hypnosis. It's totally safe and you're in total control. Remember when doing past life viewing, that you are not reliving the situation; you are only viewing it to identify and heal issues.

It's important to cleanse your energy before proceeding with any of these methods to ensure that there's no interference from anything other than what is truly you. It's also a good idea to identify and know within yourself that you want to heal past life issues.

AT': Don't flinch away, since doing so just prolongs your karmic problems. If you feel fearful, wrap your fear and hesitation in pure light and send it outward to the True Creator or Archangel Michael to clear your way forward. President John F. Kennedy once said, "The only thing to fear is fear itself," but I say, "The only thing waiting beyond the fear is the joy of healing growth." Besides, it could be that your fear is not your own, but that of an ALP which was born during the creation of the karmic issue, or maybe an intruder hiding beneath the karmic crud who knows that cleansing will reveal its hiding place or perhaps an inner child who needs healing and reclaiming. Either way, they need to be dealt with for you to heal.

Remember also that you have grown beyond who you were in these past lives. You are yourself now, regardless of what is shown in a past life. That other self used to be you, but you are much more than it now. So, if something turns up which makes you ashamed of who you were then, see it as a chance to heal that part of you, and release the shame, since it only hinders you. In the same manner, if you see a past life in which you were rich and famous, or even royalty, that isn't who you are now, and it reduces the experience of good things about that life, about any life you might glimpse. You are yourself now, and the past should only add textures and flavors to yourself, not cause you harm.

Methods for Retrieving Past Life Issues:
Method 1: Life Guide Assistance

GM: For this method, ask your life guide, or whoever is appropriate, to show you a past life that requires healing. Then trust what you see, feel, or hear and acknowledge the feelings the scene evokes. The acknowledgement and identification of those feelings are the keys to healing that life. Once you've done that, proceed to "Steps for Healing Past Life Issues" below.

Method 2: The Fishing Pole

GM: Visualize a fishing pole in your hand. Cast the line, then reel it in until you snag something. What you catch may be a scene from the past, a symbol requiring deciphering, or a sensation manifesting somewhere in your body. Once again, acknowledge the situation or item on your line including the emotions it evokes. Then proceed to "Steps for Healing Past Life Issues" below.

Method 3: The River of Time

GM: The River of Time is also known as the Akashic Record and the Tapestry of Time. They are all perspectives of the same thing, so don't be intimidated by them. Choose which perspective you feel most comfortable with, and get to know it. Through these, you can learn your soul's history, as well as your genetic history, by focusing on one or the other. If you search your genetic history, don't be concerned if you aren't able to discover "who you were," since these are your ancestors and you may or may not be among them. While it's true that we can incarnate within our own family, most souls move to other genetic lines and places to learn new lessons.

This method uses the river of time to explore our past. Visualize yourself sitting on the bank of the river of time. Look up the river until you see something. Again, appropriately acknowledge the situation and the emotions it evokes. Then proceed to "Steps for Healing Past Life Issues" below.

AT': If you see fish swimming or jumping in the river, it's a sign that past life issues are at the surface and ready to be dealt with. Use the fishing pole method to catch them before seeking deeper ones. If the river appears deep or boiling with rapids, it's a sign that your subconscious mind may fear that your consciousness is not yet ready to view or deal with these karmic issues. Ask the Holy Spirit if it is appropriate for you to proceed at this time. If it is, then ask the Holy Spirit to remove those parts of you which are fighting your growth, calve them away from you as ALPs to clear the way for healing and grow.

By following the river to its source, you may come upon a large body of water with fifteen whirlpools. These whirlpools are the fifteen time rounds that preceded the one we are now in. Sooner or later, you will have to delve into them to clear away the karmic stains they contain. Do not fear doing this, since you will always return to the here and now. Here is where you are anchored, so here is where you will always return.

Where you approach the river is now, and the past is towards its source, but you can also glance at future possibilities by looking towards the river's mouth. If you do this, however, remember that the future is only possibilities and probabilities which have not yet come into form; they change with every choice we make along the way.

So explore the possibilities of the future, but do so with the idea of seeing them as the aftermath of choices we have made or are about to make, not as something set in stone.

Steps for Healing Past Life Issues

GM: Healing past life issues is similar to the emotional release described in earlier chapters. Remember that you are not reliving past life events, but viewing them for the purpose of healing. Throughout this whole process, call on your Core Self to rise up in strength, and overflow yourself with appropriate core energies.

1. Know that all emotions from the life presenting itself are held in your emotions eyesglasses.
2. Identify, as best you can, the other people involved in the situation. If you have trouble recognizing someone, looking into their eyes may help.
3. Forgive those who have caused you to feel whatever emotions are held in your emotions eyeglasses.
4. Forgive yourself for allowing others to make you feel the emotions you are feeling, and for not trusting yourself and the life process.
5. For purposes of clearing karma, ask for all appropriate forgiveness related to the situation. There may not seem to be a reason to ask forgiveness, but it doesn't hurt, and can only benefit you in case there's some hidden reason that you need forgiveness.
6. Once forgiveness is complete, wrap the whole situation in appropriate core energies, including all emotions eyeglasses and hand all to Archangel Michael to deal with appropriately.
7. Call on the Holy Spirit to deal appropriately with all ALPs and karmic remnants.
8. Ask Archangel Michael to double-check that nothing is hiding between you and your children, as well as beneath or within any residue.
9. Call on Archangel Raphael to clear all body energy residue and all else he deems appropriate.
10. Call on the pure light vacuum to recycle all crud and miscellaneous appropriate.

Karma, Pre-Life Lessons, or Pathway Choices

AT': When cycles keep appearing in your life, they can indicate karmic attachments, pre-life lessons, or pathway choices you need to make. Karmic attachments bind you to other people because of things that caused either debit or credit involving a wounding of the soul, either yours or those bound to you.

An example of this is a woman who meets and marries a man she is instantly attracted to, who abuses her, yet she can't walk away from him. Perhaps she was the abuser in a past life and so remains until the debt is paid, or it could be that she was also abused in a previous life, and somehow feels at fault because she was unable to change her partner. Forgiving and asking forgiveness releases the debt, but individuals remain together until one or the other examines the past to see why they are still bound together. It could be the abused wife still believes she can change her husband, something out of her control. No one can change another person. Because change comes from within, you can only change yourself.

Lessons come from either past lives or pre-life choices. These are things you need to learn and acknowledge before your soul can grow towards its next stage of development. Past life lessons often involve karmic ties to others, but not always. When dealing with a past life situation, if you've released all credit and debit, examined the situation acknowledging your part in it, and are still unable to move beyond it, then there is a lesson involved which needs to be found and examined to see if you have learned it without acknowledging it.

If the lesson was a pre-life choice involving something you came to this life to learn, then deal with it in the same manner as you would past life lessons. Examine the events to which you keep cycling back, and see why you repeatedly make the same choices. Then ask your Core Self or Guardian Angel to confirm or deny whether you've recognized the lessons you are being confronted with. If you recognize them, think about the choices you make when confronting these situations and their outcomes. Understand these choices are not allowing you to learn your lesson, since the situation keeps recycling. What other choices could you make? Think. Don't be afraid to run alternate choices by your

Core Self or Guardian Angel before the event recycles. How else will you know which choice will lead to your learning the lesson? Perhaps, by reviewing your other choices, the truth of the lesson will become clear and the situation won't come up again.

An example of such a lesson is when a woman routinely chooses abusive partners. How many times have you heard a woman say, "I always end up with a man who cheats on me," or "Why do I always choose men who beat me?" It could be that each of these men is bound to this woman because of karma from abusive past lives, but it's more likely that the woman keeps recycling the situation because of a lesson she's being confronted with, but not learning. Perhaps the lesson is simply that she's worthy of being loved without the pain, or maybe that she has no need of a partner, or maybe the type of partner she needs in order to grow is the kind of man she refuses to consider as a potential mate. Think. Ask. Grow.

Pathway choices are set in your way by your future self, who can see farther ahead than your conscious mind can, it creates situations which lead you down the path you need to take to be ready for future events. When these choices aren't made, the path isn't taken, it's no big deal, since your future self has left plenty of time to make the correct choice, and the situation keeps recycling until you finally do. Your future self knows that you'll eventually catch on, either in this life or the next, so it patiently allows you the time you need.

Examples of this can be found in movies and books where two people are drawn together, yet reject that attraction for fear of losing their friendship. When they finally do come together, their lives are filled with more joy than they believed possible. Another example is if you keep choosing the same type of job, but are unhappy, or perhaps let go by the company you work for. Perhaps your future self is trying to tell you that you're not doing the kind of work you need to do. Search your heart. Ask your Core Self or Guardian Angel if there's something else you should be doing. If your Core Self or Guardian Angel don't supply the answer, listen to your heart. What type of work are you drawn to? Once you recognize the desire, ask again. Your Core Self and Guardian Angel are more likely to answer with simple yes or no responses.

The steps along your pathway are your choice, and your future self may see where you will eventually end up, but how you get there is anchored in the free will of who you are *now*. Personally, I'd like to get there as quickly and painlessly as possible. When we fight the choices and changes our future self indicates, we find fear is at the root of our avoidance; fear of change, fear of the unknown, fear of trusting our Core Self to guide us into joy. Move past the fear and reach for your future willingly, instead of fighting the changes that are trying to guide you in the right direction. The choice is yours.

Chapter 7:
Centering and Getting to Know Self

You Apart from Others

AT': As you have gone through the previous chapters you've learned how to clear away that which is not you, and what hinders your true pathway. In this chapter, I wish to reinforce that the true you can't be removed by any cleansing process, and how you can more easily identify what is truly you. People who are born empaths (see below) find it hard to tell what is truly them, apart from what they feel touching them from the outside.

Even some who are born telepaths (see below) have trouble distinguishing between their own thoughts, and thoughts they receive from others. Most of the world's population have some form of telepathic or empathic abilities, but don't recognize their abilities. With practice, you can learn the difference between your own thoughts or feelings and those of others.

Regions within Self

AT': No matter what names you give to the portions of your self, they are all still you and you have free will to choose which regions to ponder. Higher self, highest self, inner self, Core Self (Appendix 10) are all names we give to regions within us (Appendices 3, 4). They act to reduce the stress on our material minds as we access deeper knowing or find new talents. When you call on certain parts of yourself for information or confirmation, it is the intent and need behind your call that draws forth these regional parts of yourself. The parts you call, regardless of the names you use, will be the appropriate ones to support you, even if you can't feel or hear them—after all, they are you.

You are always in charge, the one who owns your body by right of being born into it through your pre-life choices while in the realms of light, and by the weight of your karmic ties to the family and circumstances you were born into. Don't get confused; it comes down to the simple statement I am. Claim all you are and all you were born to be, during this lifetime and by the pathway the True Creator birthed you to evolve into.

When we were newborns at the beginning of time, the True Creator gave each of us a core of power which included all of the below:

1. A template of the First Dream's paradox of time (see Appendix 11), from each individual's perspective within that dream. This is also called your true facet self.

2. A template of our dream body's DNA for us to grow into.

3. A true jobs list which echoes the dream template, revealing things for us to do or help with in manifesting the paradox of time (Appendix 9) to see what lies beyond.

4. A hunger that leads us down our true pathway to our individual places within the paradox of time, bringing it full circle. Even when we stray from our path or take a vacation from it, the hunger for more always brings us back.

5. Free will to choose our individual footsteps along our path, since only then can we achieve our fullest potential, evolving into who we were born to be.

6. Your core, which protects all these things and the true you. Nothing can penetrate this except Archangel Michael's weapons of pure light, and then only when you give permission. The True Creator has no need to penetrate your core's shield since He/She is the force holding it all together. (See below for details regarding false cores.)

Another part of self you need to be aware of is your future self; who you are growing into within this particular lifetime. If part of your future self awakens within you before its time, perhaps there are bindings around it interfering with your growth. This is especially troubling when it occurs in a child, seemingly possessed by an intruder or a dominant ALP, but none of the cleansings work. The only way to deal with a prematurely awakened future self is to call the pure light to shatter the barrier between the self of now and the future self. Once that barrier is shattered, call upon the Core Self to wrap the future self in unconditional love and a fantasy bubble, and send it to sleep until it is time for it to awaken.

False Cores

AT': False cores are something you need to be aware of and eventually dissolve. In an attempt to bind your memories, scars, and other things which hindered you, false cores were created around your true core when each of the fifteen time rounds imploded, so you could begin the new time round clean and whole. This didn't work, because false cores leak. Memories, curses, spells, etc. spill over into the present. Why? Because we're following the same pathway towards the First Dream's True United Destiny. As we intertwine with others doing the same, similar situations occur which force old memories to the surface, causing us to repeat old choices, and warping us away from possible new choices and actions.

How to tell if the memory that has surfaced is from this timeline or leaking from a false core can be tricky without experience, but they do feel different. If you've delved into your past lives or early memories from this life, you know their feel, but those from other time rounds have a different texture and flavor to them. You could even say they have a stale taste since they are from dead time, time no longer flowing as the time we are now surrounded by is. Another clue to ancient time memories may be the images themselves. They may appear similar to that which has occurred in our present timeline, but there will be differences. For example, we used horses and wagons for travel near home, but hovercrafts for distant journeys. Many stories we find in books labeled as fiction are such memories leaking past false cores, such as the stories of King Arthur and Merlin, and even the *Lord of the Rings* saga. Pay attention to the details of the memories to place them in their proper time period. If you find ancient memories surfacing before you've cleared away the false cores, it's a sign that you may be ready to begin.

Everything you have previously cleared away must be repeated in stripping away false cores. Many of you may have thought you were accessing core information, or think you're balanced within your Core Self.

Try this: ask your Guardian Angels or guides to turn and see the teachers and guides willing to teach them previously unknown truths about past time rounds. Then ask them if it is time to begin dismantling the false cores. If the answer is *Yes*, follow the commands below, remembering that there are fifteen false cores and they must be removed individually.

1. Call on the pure light quicksilver to ignite in and around the false core, begin dissolving it, and vacuuming it up from the inside out and the outside in.

2. Ask Archangel Michael, the Holy Spirit, and all others appropriate to find and deal with everything hidden in and beneath the false core. Be prepared to repeat any of the cleansing commands found in previous chapters, since those doing the cleansing must be sure you truly want all of it removed.

3. Don't be surprised if memories that need to be faced and healed surface from other time rounds.

4. Give yourself time to rebalance and absorb what you need to reclaim in the space once taken up by the false core.

5. As you proceed, ask your guides to tell you what percentage of the false core is dissolved, and how much of what was hidden has been dealt with. Continue to do this until you receive the answer that nothing is left.

6. Once you have cleared away the false core and dealt with everything beneath it, repeat the process for the other false cores.

Remember all fifteen false cores need to be dealt with individually, and you may need time between each to fully absorb them. Be patient. It takes time to reclaim those parts of you that have been uncovered.

Once you've cleared away all fifteen of your false cores, go to Chapter 8 and follow the directions for reclaiming your inner core. If you've already done this, humor me and do it again, noting the difference in what you feel or see now that your false cores have been dealt with.

Source of Thoughts

AT': Learn the difference between yourself and outsiders. Recognize the thoughts you hear or feel within and discern their origin. Note that it takes practice to recognize the texture and flavor of different voices. Don't be afraid of asking for the source of the thoughts you hear within your mind. (Appendix 2 has a list of outsiders.)

Below is a list of the most dominant sources of thoughts and where you will hear their voices. Their locations are the same in everyone, although you may find other areas of your brain echoing the thoughts of other parts of yourself or outsiders. Always ask until you become familiar enough with them to identify them by their texture and feel.

1. Future Self: The you of the First Dream's template, heard in the front of the brain, in the top left corner.

2. Mitochondrial (Mito's) Mind: The symbionts found in each cell of our body that we can't live without; our partners and companions throughout life. These are heard as one being at the base of the skull. When asked, they will give you a name, which is the opposite gender to your own. Although their physical form is given to you by your mother, their souls come with you into the flesh and leave with you when the flesh dies.

3. Ancestral Mind: Sometimes calling themselves the Old Ones, their voice comes to us in the right temple near the forehead through our DNA and gives us access to our ancestors. Note that ALPs are also heard in this location.

4. Outsider Spirits: These are the voices of life guides, Guardian Angels, Archangels, and other outsiders including lost souls, souls who are in the light, and spirits of all kinds outside yourself. They are heard in or around the right ear.

5. Outsider Flesh-bound: These are animals and people in flesh, whose voices are heard through the center of the forehead, the third-eye area and higher.

6. Spiritual Mind: These symbionts are intertwined with your limbic system and throat, and tuned to your body in order to help you stay healthy. This voice is heard just to the right of the mitochondrial voice at the base of the brain, but it won't give you a name for itself as the mitos do, since they are born with and die with your flesh.

7. Analytical Mind: These symbionts are tuned to the left side of your brain and help keep you balanced here in the material world.

They are heard just to the left of the mitochondrial voice at the base of the brain and also refuse to think of themselves as separate from you since they, too, are bound to the flesh and die with it.

8. Elemental Entities: These spirits have more substance than angels and less than us here in flesh. They are bound to the regions of the earth and are sometimes called Earth Spirits, dealing mainly with rooted and growing things. They also tend to the ley lines, Earth's energy flows, and enjoy interacting with us when we recognize them. They can be heard around the left ear area of the brain.

9. Me/I: This is the you who owns the material body and has conscious choice. It is the unification of all other parts of the self, even if you don't recognize all these parts that intertwine. It is heard at the center of the brain.

10. Creatures: These are the creatures of mythology, i.e. sprites, fairies, leprechauns, griffons, centaurs, dragons (not Baks' shape-changer ones), merpeople, etc. A thin veil that they can easily cross separates their world from ours. They love interacting with us. You can hear them in the left temple area of the brain.

11. False Beings: These are creations that duplicate real spirits, but were set in place to lead you in directions their creators wished you to go. They can be heard either near the right or left ears, but can be hard to discern from real beings. The best way to tell the difference is to wrap them in unconditional love and pure light and ask Archangels Michael and Azrael to deal with them appropriately. If they are false beings, they will vanish. If they are real beings, they will simply smile and enjoy the cleansing without offence.

Don't worry about offending angels or others by asking their names and jobs, since those who are appropriately there for your highest good are eager to ease your concerns by answering. If they don't answer, or you continue to feel uneasy, call on Archangel Michael or Archangel Gabriel to talk to them and see that all which is appropriate occurs. If you're dealing with internal thoughts or feelings, ask the Holy Spirit to stand by to take any and all ALPs which might be uncovered during your inward explorations.

Are You Empathic or Telepathic?

AT': Are you empathic? Do you sometimes suddenly feel pain that doesn't last? How about intense emotions that don't relate to your present circumstances? True depression, whether manic or otherwise, has a definite affect on your body's chemistry, but with empathetic individuals it leaves the body's chemistry unaltered because it is received from outside.

Try the first thought technique. Ask yourself, "Is this my pain or emotion, or am I receiving this from an outside source?" If its source is your own, seek out a doctor or psychologist to help you. If the source is external, ask if it is appropriate for you to be feeling it. If it isn't appropriate, rebirth your personal shields and demand that Archangels Raphael and Michael deal with the source and block it from you. If it is appropriate for you to feel it, perhaps you have the ability to help whoever is in pain. Ask the soul who you are receiving from what they need from you. If you don't receive an answer, it could mean a few things. Try asking yes or no questions, such as, "Do I personally know the person I am receiving from?" If *Yes*, then ask specific names until you receive confirmation. Silence could also indicate that you are receiving from a lost soul who has been drawn to you because of your sensitivity. Ask, "Is the one I am receiving from in flesh or in spirit?" If in spirit, ask, "Have they been to the light?" If the answer is *No*, then call on Archangel Michael to guide them to the light. Even if they have a message they wish you to deliver, how can they clearly communicate their message if they haven't yet been healed by the light?

GM: Spirits that haven't been to the light yet for healing, haven't been for various reasons; the main one is that they fear being judged, and not being worthy of and accepted in heaven, based on their perception of mistakes made in their life, or various beliefs. Lost spirits are stuck and have their earthly baggage and emotions. It is important for them to have the opportunity to heal and continue their growth. A wonderful tool you can set up to help lost spirits and gain some control over your experiences with spirits, is the building of pure light, as described below:

1.   Visualize a building of pure light with two rooms.
2.   The first room is for lost spirits to be directed to by your guide. When the lost spirit enters this room they will automatically be wrapped in a blanket of unconditional love and undiluted joy, a pure light vacuum tunnel will be set up, and all appropriate loved ones in the light will come to meet them.
3.   The second room is a place for spirits that have been to the light to sit and wait until you are able to help them connect with loved ones.
4.   Once the building is complete, ask your appropriate guide to direct all spirits to the appropriate rooms.
5.   There may be an opportunity in which, due to intense emotions, the lost spirit will require extra attention to go to the light. In these cases, once wrapped in unconditional love, simply and lovingly encourage them to look to the tunnel you have created for them with their loved ones, and explain to them that they can return at will, once they have been to the light. Also, it is important they understand that no one will be judging them or their life. All are welcome and it is a joyous time when they return to the light.

AT': Telepathy is similarly dealt with by asking the who, what, when, where, and why of the thoughts you hear. Whose voice it is can be narrowed down by noticing where the thoughts originate in your mind (see list in "Source of Thoughts" above), since to me telepathy and clairaudience (hearing spirit) are just flipsides of the same coin. By noting where the voice is heard, you know whether you're dealing with someone in flesh or spirit. If you hear thoughts in the center of your forehead, you're listening to one in flesh, so ask first if their conscious mind is aware they are sending you their thoughts. If you get a *No*, then ask if it is appropriate for you to be hearing these thought projections. If you still get a *No*, ask your personal shields to "rebirth and block this person's sending without hindering appropriate communications." If the answer to either question is *Yes*, then ask why you are hearing them. It could be that you are hearing family or friends, or even someone who is seeking guidance that you can give them, soul to soul, so ask what their need is. If what you are hearing is something negative or damaging to you, or you simply don't wish to receive from that person, then rebirth your shields as stated above, refining the shields by continuing to rebirth them until they block the unwanted thoughts from others. If dealing with those in spirit, another good question to ask is when their voices are originating, since thoughts are energy and can bounce around the universe and beyond for ages until they thump into someone's mind and are absorbed. If the voices are from now, ask questions similar to those above to decide if it's appropriate for you to be hearing them. As with empathic feelings, if you receive thoughts from a soul who has not yet been to the light, these thoughts may be chaotic and hard to understand, so ask Archangel Michael to gather them in and take them to the light, letting the spirit know (if you choose) that they can return when they have been healed in the light. What sets telepathy apart from schizophrenia is the brain chemistry, since a telepath's chemistry is normal.

Other things to remember about either telepathic or empathic touch is that it can be helpful to yourself or others, or it can be a distraction hindering you from walking your true pathway. Keep this in mind as you ask your questions.

Future Self, Soul History, and Genetic History

AT': Who you are today is a combination of what you have experienced from the time of your birth from the True Creator, who you are growing into, and what your body's genetics allow you to bring into this lifetime.

Who you are growing into is your future self, the you of the True Creator's First Dream True United Destiny born from it. This part of yourself has a great influence over what choices open to you as you walk your pathway, since it sees things from the perspective of the future. It is very patient since it knows you have plenty of time to grow into your self, but it is also persistent, continually setting before you options for the path you need to follow. One way your future self might be trying to direct you is in the job market or education. A woman I know went to college for many years, taking courses in languages and commerce. She wished to continue her education, gathering higher degrees, but kept flunking out. Once she decided to stop her schooling, she quickly got hired in her field of expertise and began to put that knowledge to work. By flunking out of her classes, her future self was trying to tell her to go and live life now and not wait, that she already had what she needed.

Your genetic heritage is also important in that it provides your material roots on the planet. It is the culmination of thousands of generations before you, evolving humanity towards the True United Destiny we all share. This unites all genetic lines to form a magnificent moment in time when humanity will help bring together all telepathic races in the galaxy bringing the paradox of time, which birthed the First Dream, full circle. You and your family are helping by giving your progeny the chance to be there at the nanosecond of the First Dream manifesting. As was stated in the "Regions Within Self," we each have DNA coded in our Core Self and the genetic lines of earth are evolving towards those future bodies we will need.

Your soul's history is who you were in and between all your past lives, and who you are growing into today. Memories from those past lives give you the textures and flavors that make you an individual now. Some memories may be scars or unhealed wounds that need to be dealt with using the exercises in the other chapters. Healed or unhealed, these add to who you are. You would not be who you are now without them.

GM: An example of this is a friend of ours who went through some horrendous events in her life, and has now begun to recognize a strength deep within, one that has helped her realize a sense of love of self that was always there, but hidden by other emotions.

AT': Together, they have all shaped the you of today, the you the True Creator needs you to be. It is this person who has reached for this book to help you grow into who you will become in the future. Rejoice in who you are. The True Creator does.

Chapter 8:
Expanding Boundaries
of Thought and Self

Why Expand Self and Boundaries?

AT': Once you are clean of outside influences, harmful emotions, and karmic crud, it's time to understand who you truly are and why you're here. To do that, you must realize that you are more than flesh, more than your place in society and in family, more than who you think you are. The first step in doing this is reclaiming your inner core, which helps you reclaim all the particles that anchor you within existence. The next step is finding and removing all false beliefs, deceptions, false knowledge, false perceptions, false perspectives, self-deceptions, wrongful oaths, and preconceptions which hinder you from being able to see the truth behind the truth of yourself, all else, and all others. In this chapter are several exercises to help you do this, and although they appear simple and superficially may seem like things others have told you to do, in truth they are difficult because you must persevere and fight to strip away things you may have been clinging to as anchors. I promise you that new and better anchors will appear.

GM: By this point in the book, you have been busy working on self, and the more you do it, the deeper you will get. You may find yourself feeling anger and frustration, impatience with the whole process of growth and healing. As with all uncomfortable feelings you may experience in doing Wild Card therapy, it is a clue to you that what you are feeling is something hindering your growth and healing; for example, clinging to something that your Core Self knows not to be true, yet not having explored it consciously to understand or reject it. In working with people, I've come across many situations in which those I'm working with have become antagonistic, not to me personally, but in general. In most cases, the source of that antagonism was their holding onto a belief that isn't conducive to taking responsibility for their own feelings and actions.

There was a deep-seated fear of not being good enough as a person. Some have felt anger, frustration, and guilt, at the idea of allowing themselves to grow and heal. Many share the idea that doing for self or taking care of self is selfish and that we should only help others. In identifying and rejecting this falsehood, we are able to see that taking care of self is a necessity, allowing everything in relation to helping and doing for others to fall into place. Once you give yourself permission to let go, you will find yourself much calmer and more content. In cases where there are things about you that you have been told are not acceptable, yet you feel an understanding and acceptance of, embrace those things as being a part of you rather than continuing on with the inner battle. Identifying and understanding is your key to growing joyfully.

Reclaiming Your Inner Core

AT': The Wild Cards of the Ivory Tower, Command Center, and Control Room are helpful in reclaiming your inner core. Don't worry if the cards you see in your mind's eye don't look exactly like those drawn on the Wild Cards, since each is as individual as your soul. These are short cuts to seeking your core, saving time when you try to find the deepest part of yourself. This is the source of inner knowing, the birthplace of your personal shields, the part of you which can only be accessed by the true you, the True Creator and Archangel Michael's sword of pure light. Make sure you have done the Chapter 7 exercises before continuing with this chapter.

GM: A woman I was working with to reclaim her command center had an interesting and insightful experience. In activating the Ivory Tower Wild Card, she saw a stairway leading to its top. She followed the stairs up, wrapping all that caused her to have any feelings of fear, anger, or hesitation until she reached the pinnacle. At the top, she saw a hallway with two doors. She opened the first door where she saw a bench, rather than a chair. She saw a bench because she was sharing the command of herself with others. In other words, she wasn't prepared to take full control and responsibility for herself. The bench was wrapped up, yet stayed. Realizing that a bench is inappropriate to reclaiming your own command center, we went through the next door to see if we could identify what was hindering her. In the second room, she saw her grandmother and other relatives who had already passed. It turned out that as a result of their belief systems, these loved ones were actually stuck in a place they believed to be heaven, when in fact they hadn't yet gone to the light. Once we wrapped them up in a fantasy teaching bubble and called on appropriate teachers and guides, her loved ones learned of the hindrance of their beliefs, and willingly went to the light. Now that the second room was dealt with, we returned to the first room to find the bench had changed into a chair. Having dealt with her relatives' beliefs freed her from the bindings passed on to her from those beliefs, and to take appropriate responsibility and control of her command center.

To reclaim your inner core, activate the Wild Cards and then follow the steps below.

1. Focus on the Ivory Tower (seen on the cover) and picture it directly in front of you. Ask the Holy Spirit and Archangel Michael to stand by to take any and everything that is not truly you.

2. Climb to the top of the Tower and enter the flower-shaped Command Center that coordinates your parts and particles.

3. Walk to the center of the Command Center, where the Control Room sphere is waiting for you to reclaim it.

4. Step into the Control Room and sit in the chair waiting at its center. Feel it solidly beneath you. Feel the chair wrap itself around you and remember that it is you.

5. Now open yourself to it, draw it into you, meld with it. By becoming the chair, you reclaim the Control Room, which links you to every part and particle of your body.

6. Note, but do not be concerned by, the sensations you feel in various parts of your body as you tune yourself to the chair. These feelings are either your growing awareness of parts of yourself which have been closed off, or they are Archangel Michael and the Holy Spirit removing that which is not you, including ALPs which are calving away from you as you grow.

7. Once you've tuned yourself to the chair's powers and feel comfortable,

call on the chair-that-is-you to grow outward, claiming all your parts and particles, expanding outward to your outermost particles in existence. Remember that you can't grow beyond your outermost particle; growth is limited to the whole of your greater self.

8.   Once your outward growth has stopped, call on Archangel Michael and the Holy Spirit to do a thorough cleansing of all your parts and particles and between, since these newly recovered parts of you may have things overlapping them, which could hinder them settling into place.

9.   Now relax and explore the greater you. You may find you need to reject falsehoods and preconceptions before you fully open to the whole of yourself, but now you have a solid and true anchor to balance your growth.

Creator's Laundry Chute

AT': Now that you have reclaimed your inner core, it may be the right time to reclaim your access to the True Creator that resides within your core. This is a simple process if you visualize that access point as a laundry chute through which you can flush out all the crud and emotional residue hindering you, releasing it to the True Creator who recycles it through pure light. Visualize this chute with two-way access; the True Creator can take that which you release to Him and He can return unconditional love and other refined powers to you, filling all the places emptied.

GM: An interesting example of using the laundry chute came quite early on in the process of developing Wild Card therapy. At that time, I chatted quite regularly with a woman who, unbeknownst to me, had multiple personalities. I only discovered this when one of the multiples surfaced as we were chatting one day. This multiple was aged sixteen and protecting another who was a child of five. In chatting with this multiple, we spoke of many things including love, which was an unheard of concept to her. She only knew pain and considered herself protective of the woman. It was difficult to explain love to someone who had absolutely no concept of it, but she could understand when we spoke about pain. She agreed after much discussion to use the laundry chute to eject the pain she was holding onto for the woman. It was amazing to me how she felt a difference after having gone through the exercise, and was willing and wanting to go with Archangel Michael for help.

Since that experience, we've learned a lot about multiple personalities. They appear to be a combination of ALPs and inner(s) that needs reclaiming (see Chapter 5). We have encountered various situations, since this example, of people who controlled the use of their multiples. For instance, one woman I worked with was very aware of her multiples, and called them into action at various times. If something came up that she didn't want to deal with, she'd call on the multiple she felt would deal with it best, and she would step back. She worked very hard in healing those memories that had created the multiples in the first place, and has found that she isn't able to access the multiples anymore because she has healed and reclaimed those parts of herself. In being able to reclaim those parts of herself, she found she was allowing her true self to feel and become able to deal with and heal those feelings that at one time she would have called upon a fractured part of herself to deal with.

To access the Creator's Laundry Chute:

1. Visualize your inner core and look at its centermost point.
2. At that center, visualize a trapdoor.
3. Open the trapdoor and push out all the crud; all the old essence, emotional residue, and anything else that doesn't have awareness pieces in it. Push it all through the trapdoor and down the chute, releasing it to the True Creator for recycling.
4. Now, visualize the chute made of pure light quicksilver. As you push out the trash, the Creator is automatically returning to you all the energy and love you need through the material of the chute itself.
5. Continue releasing all the crud until there's nothing left to be taken. As you do so, ask the Holy Spirit and Archangel Michael to clear away any ALPs and others who have been clinging or hiding.
6. Once everything has been released, ask your Core Self and the pure light quicksilver to reclaim and rebalance all places emptied.

Remember, you can see God in others around you, but when you try to access God through them, you only get their version of God. Like looking through a window, you'd never be able to touch God intimately that way. It's only when you access God, the True Creator, through your own inner core that you can know Him intimately.

Shifting Balance Anchors

AT': Sometimes, when you are growing, you realize there are things that must be cleared to continue that growth. You may have to shift your mental anchors to move forward. This happens when what must be stripped away is clinging to false beliefs, or other thought processes, on which you have relied. The Holy Spirit, or others working on you, may fear you might become unbalanced when these falsehoods are stripped away and they won't remove anything for fear of harming you. Once you find a new, solid anchor, unattached to these falsehoods, they will continue their cleansing.

I can't choose your anchor for you, but I can tell you about my own, that which has allowed me to rip away falsehoods, while remaining free and balanced as knowledge has shifted into new and true shapes. In Appendix 11, I speak of the True Creator's First Dream, and in Appendix 12, I list my beliefs, born of my anchoring to the First Dream and my perspective within the First Dream template at my core. Stating it another way, I am anchored to my true pathway leading to my place and perspective within that First Dream. Everyone has their own perspective of the First Dream that no one else can share, since each being, in and beyond existence, was born to recreate the individuals within that First Dream.

Know that everything you have experienced has led you to where you are now, even if that place has fought against your true pathway; each step was needed to shape you into who you are and prepare you for moving forward. That doesn't mean you should continue to fight your true pathway into the First Dream, but what has come before this has prepared you to grasp what is to come and allow you to understand the unique pieces of truths you hold within your inner core. Don't be concerned that embracing your perspective within the First Dream's template will cause problems in your family life, unless those problems already exist, since your family is part of your true pathway. If you are concerned, ask your guides or inner core to see if your growth will move you away from your family, if your growth will help your family grow as well, or if the problems you encounter in your family are because you don't belong among them. It could be, as with many married couples, that you were drawn together to learn certain lessons, and when those lessons are learned, you move on; or perhaps in growing you will inspire your partner to grow, so both of you will reach for new lessons to learn together.

To shift your anchor to your perspective within the First Dream, follow these steps:

1. Focus on your chair in the Control Room of your Ivory Tower. Open yourself to your innate perspective within the First Dream, and know that the template of the First Dream surrounds you while you are seated here.

2. Now say these words, or words with this intent: "I reject any anchor except that which opens me to the truth behind the truth of myself, and my place within the First Dream, so that I may choose my steps truly as I walk my true pathway into the First Dream."

3. Call on Archangel Michael to stand between you and everyone or everything hindering your growth, even if they are doing so out of concern for you. Remember, this includes all who are outside you, as well as that which is within you.

4. Ask the Holy Spirit to remove any and all ALPs which have calved away from you, and also those that have not yet calved away, yet are rejecting your growth. You have the right to grow and if anyone or anything is hindering that process, you have the right to demand their removal.

Ways to Reject What Hinders Truth

AT': What follows are examples of power words and exercises and how they can be used to cut through to the truth buried within yourself. This is the part that appears simple, and yet is difficult. You may have been told about the power of words, but not how to use them for guidance in stripping away deceptions and other such hindrances to the truth. These words are used as a power focus or method of emptying your head, but here they are used to access what is in your head, heart, and past. The power words aren't set in stone, but these examples will help guide you until you feel confident enough in your inner knowing to create your own power words.

The power words are repeated over and over again, either aloud or silently, until thoughts or visions intrude with information you need to discover the truth buried within you. You might only have to say them a few times before a vision or thought rises up, but don't worry if you have to repeat them many times, especially when you first begin reaching for the truth. If the words change, notice how this transition changes the meaning or intent of the words. If the changes take you away from what you're seeking, ask the Holy Spirit or Archangel Michael to deal with the intruders or ALPs which may be fighting your reaching for the truth.

If the changes sharpen the focus on what you're seeking, use that change to help cut through the crud in your search for the truth. Remember, what you find may be the reason you believe in things which are hiding the truth, why you flinch away from the truth in favor of a comforting falsehood, or perhaps it's simply that you fear the truth will invalidate your life up to this point. The truth is that anything or anyone who hides the truth from you isn't working for your highest good; even if the truth is painful in the beginning, no falsehood can help you grow. Your life has been what you needed it to be until now, to grow to the point of being ready for the truth.

In the following sections are various power words and exercises, and discussions regarding why you need to strip away these things to see the truth of who you are and who you are growing into. Remember, the only way the truth can cause you lasting harm is if you refuse to see and embrace it. Only by accepting the truth, no matter how painful, can you grow into who the True Creator birthed you to become.

GM: By definition, power words can be taken as a mantra or chant. To ensure there are no preconceptions or false perceptions created from others' meanings of these terms, we have chosen the term "power words."

Seeking the Truth Behind the Truth

AT': In my own growth, I have found that the truth is only a starting place, since there are many layers of truth that add up to a greater truth. Also, if you're conversing with someone, watching TV or a movie, and either flinch away from something you see or hear, or feel drawn to it, it usually indicates something you should delve farther into. I've also discovered that as much as angels and the hierarchies of light know, they don't know everything. They know only those areas of truth dealing with their own regions of knowledge and existence, which is the same for most of us here in the flesh.

I don't claim to know everything either, and hope to always find new things to learn and grow into. Here are the power words I began growing with, using them to learn how to recognize truth from falsehood in what I come upon here on earth and out beyond the material:

> "I seek the truth, and the truth behind the truth of myself, all else, and all others which I am ready to understand even as I reject all that hinders the truth."

Keys and Gateways

AT': Another way of expanding yourself is to see truths as keys to gateways buried deep within yourself holding even more truth. Each person holds pieces of the truth within themselves, which may appear contradictory to those others hold, but when all the pieces are fitted together, they form a greater truth. Think of truth as a shattered crystal with each person holding a shard. All the pieces are needed to see the whole crystal, just as each piece of truth is needed to see the greater truth.

GM: A common example of this is the voices or thoughts you have. Your awareness of self and openness to trusting your true self will help you identify those thoughts or things you hear as not being the true you. It is those pieces of the truth within that are sparking your feeling that something doesn't sound right or sound like you.

Try this exercise:

1.   If someone tells you something that causes you to flinch away from their words, look within yourself and ask your inner core what piece of what they're saying is a truth you can grasp.

2.   Finding that piece of truth, use it as a key. Take the key and turn inward even farther, to visualize a door or gateway to your inner core.

3.   Use the key to unlock the gate, open the gate and step within.

4.   Open your heart to the truth buried within you, and draw it into every particle of your being, then allow the truth to rise up into your consciousness. Don't be concerned if what you find contradicts what the other person said. Remember, your reclaiming your own shard of the truth doesn't invalidate the other person's shard. Only when all the shards are brought together from each being can the greater whole of the subject finally be seen.

5.   End by doing the thorough cleansing from Chapter 2 to ensure nothing interferes with your reclaiming the truths buried within you.

Rejecting Falsehoods

AT': False beliefs, false knowledge, false perceptions, and false perspectives, as well as deceptions, can be hard to reject and grow beyond. You may have to rip apart what you know and reorganize it in a new way to anchor the truths within the greater whole of the truths that exist within your core and the cores of those around you. Note that perceptions and perspectives are not the same thing, perceptions being "how" and perspectives being "where" we gather the information our brains process. The words below can be modified to focus on a specific falsehood, or to call on the highest forms of light or energy rather than the True Creator, as long as the intent is clear.

> "True Creator, please help me to identify and reject
> any false belief, false knowledge, false perception,
> false perspective, or deception which hinders my
> growth or true pathway."

Once you have done this, repeat the cleansing from Chapter 2 to ensure everything is dealt with appropriately.

GM: It is important to be aware of false beings to get the full affect from Wild Card therapy. Whether or not you want to believe these exist, at least be open to the possibility, which will allow the true beings called upon in Wild Card therapy to do their jobs. False beings who claim to be any of those we call on in Wild Card Therapy don't realize they are not, because they haven't looked beyond themselves. Beliefs can create beings who, through the thought energy behind their creation, truly believe themselves to be the true beings. The problem with them is that they don't have the power to do the job that true beings have. I've been through numerous examples of a false Jesus Christ being with people. The false JC feels "right," yet when you go to do confirmations or question them to ensure their authenticity, they get upset, or don't answer questions and preach instead. The true JC has only unconditional love, which means your questioning and confirming doesn't upset him. The true being understands, whereas the false ones don't and can get quite irate. I've had many a false JC upset with me for the questions I've had others ask them. In some cases, I've been described as the devil (another being created through thought energy), or been reminded that I am loved at times when that answer didn't fit the question. The reason these beings get so upset is because they are not the true being full of unconditional love. And since Wild Card therapy and I will only deal with true beings, they will be dealt with, and I'm sure they sense their time is running out. Your best defense is to confirm with whatever beings that they are who they say they are. The confirmations you can use are those for confirming your Guardian Angel in Chapter 5.

AT': False contracts with spirit beings can be very hard to deal with, since they play on your beliefs and fears. During the Angel Wars, many dark spirits used such things to bind you to them, but they lied to get you to agree. They will never uphold their end of the contract, since it goes against your true pathway. Even if the false contract was to a light spirit, it hinders you and is harming your free will choice. Know that you have the right to shatter the contract without guilt, because you will never achieve what you need to otherwise. If you're willing to see the truth, know what the contract is, and know they have not kept their word, then follow the steps below.

1. In your own words, reject the contract (from eternity and before), and demand that it be shattered and vacuumed up in all its forms and bindings. For example, "I reject any and all false contracts, from this life and any other, which hinders me on my true pathway."

2. Ask that everyone and everything involved in any way with this false contract be wrapped in pure light quicksilver, core energies, and unconditional love.

3. Demand that those who have been attached to you because of it now be sent into the light to be cleansed, healed, and taught the truth of their wrongful actions.

4. Call on all Wild Card Therapy commands, all those appropriate to use them, and all Wild Cards and pseudo-Wild Cards (seen and unseen), to activate, and do all needed to strip the false contract away.

5. Ask that you be rebalanced with the foundations of existence, and that the area involved with the false contract be compared to the you of the First Dream template, and demand what isn't appropriate be dealt with.

6. Call on Archangel Michael and the pseudo-nephilim in the light to do all appropriate, in case they have a job to do, and repeat the exercises earlier in the book to insure all is dealt with.

Rejecting Self-Hindrances

AT': Self-deceptions, wrongful oaths or contracts, and preconceptions, are a few of those things that our conscious mind can be unaware of which hinder our growth and truth pathway. All those listed, including false promises, can follow us from lifetime to lifetime until they have been dealt with appropriately. Being unconscious, or subconsciously controlled in self-defense, these are harder impediments to recognize, which means they are that much more important to cleanse. If your subconscious mind is hiding these things from you, reassure this part of yourself that you're ready and eager for the growth that will occur once these falsehoods are stripped away. If your subconscious remains stubborn, call on the Holy Spirit and consciously calve away that part of your subconscious as an ALP. Remember, the longer you cling to these hindrances, the longer they will delay your growth along your true pathway. Here are the power words to help clear them away:

> "I ask the True Creator to help me identify and reject
> any self-deceptions, wrongful oaths, or preconceptions
> hindering my growth and true pathway."

Here again, do the thorough cleansing from Chapter 2 to clear your way for continued growth.

GM: While we may not always realize it, our thoughts and thought focus is very powerful. In situations of intense emotion, we may resort to "doing deals" with God or others to have the situation resolve as we would like it resolved. A woman I once worked with told me of her mother having a contract with "God" that she would live until her children were okay. This was a false contract. It wasn't an appropriate deal and it hindered her true pathway. The only people who truly had control over how well her children did were her children themselves. They had the free will choice to choose actions and live their consequences. Her agreement first bound her, and set up a situation in which the potential for her children's free will choice was also hindered. This false contract made with a false being (because the True Creator would never make such a deal) caused her much pain and anguish. This woman's health was failing, and on top of that was the pain and anguish from not seeing any kind of healing in her family. Clinging to this false contract created her own illnesses, intense emotions, and the waiting and wanting of her family to heal. As with all experiences, we can find a silver lining in even the worst situations that will help us grow and learn. In this particular example, although clinging to this contract caused her to linger past the exit that would have saved her and her family much pain and suffering, it also enabled our friend to help her mother heal spiritually.

Warning Signals and Calving Away What Resonates

AT': Set up a signal within yourself so you can recognize when you're facing either deception or self-deception, and can choose whether or not to embrace these. You can't stop others from attempting to deceive you, but you can change yourself so they can't affect you. Note that I ask you to do this three times, for deceptions, your self-deceptions, and others' self-deceptions, with a separate signal for each.

For example, when I'm faced with deceptions, I see a sword swinging in circles in front of me slicing away any attempts of these deceptions to bind me. When I think or say something that is a self-deception, the sword swings in circles on my right side; for self-deceptions of others, the sword swings in circles on my left. When I reach the truth behind these deceptions, and/or self-deceptions, the sword halts pointing upward in front of me. When I send forth the truth to the beings of light who work with me, the sword swings downward with its point buried in the earth at my feet.

Do not attempt the exercise below until you have reclaimed your Ivory Tower and Control Room, since then you will be able to access your Core Self. I learned this the hard way while teaching a class on this method, before teaching the Ivory Tower. One student constantly bombarded me with questions and challenges. When I sought the why of this, I found that she wasn't listening to her Core Self, but to intruders and outsiders who had been influencing her falsely for years. They were telling her that everything I said was false, when in fact they weren't allowing her to seek the truth within herself. So, first claim access to your Inner Core and then you can be confident that the answers you receive in this exercise are based in truth.

Below are the steps to creating your own warning signals. Repeat them for each of the three uses.

1. Begin by repeating: "I now call upon my Core Self and my true Guardian Angels to give me a signal, which I can recognize to warn me of deceptions (my self-deceptions, others' deceptions), both deliberate or otherwise."

2. Pay attention to what the signal is. It could be a symbol or word that flashes through your mind, a sensation or feeling, or perhaps even a smell. Whatever it is, ask your Core Self and Guardian Angels to repeat it for verification.

3. If you receive nothing, do the cleansings from the previous chapters to clear the way and repeat steps 1 and 2 until you finally know the signal.

4. Once you have this set of signals, when you receive warnings of deceptions or self-deceptions, wrap in unconditional love and appropriate energies those parts of you which resonate with the deceptions and give them to the Holy Spirit as ALPs. Ask Archangel Michael and whoever else is appropriate, to cleanse beneath where these were. Tell them to continue to strip away whatever the deception touched, since these parts are not truly you, and the true you lies beneath. Do this whenever needed.

GM: Another tool for validating the truth is the pseudo-Wild Card called the Truth Harp. When you visualize it and ask it to activate and do all appropriate, start by strumming the strings and you'll feel it resonate within you. Below are the steps for using the harp.

1. Visualize writing a statement on a piece of paper that you want to know the truth and/or appropriateness of.

2. Take the paper and run it through the strings of the harp.

3. If the paper goes through the strings without hindrance, then the statement is true or appropriate. Those pieces of paper that can't go through are shredded, declaring the statement either not truth, or inappropriate. If part of it goes through and part is shredded, try breaking the statement up and sending it through in sections. This will help you identify what is false from what is true.

Removing the Divisions Within Self

AT': Now that you've completed this book, you may find the divisions between parts of yourself are bothering you, which means it's time to get rid of most of them. Ones you can't remove are the shields around your Core Self, your shadow self, and your personal shields, since these protect you both from within and without. The reason you can't remove your Core Self's division is because they were established by the True Creator to ensure your individuality, while your Core Self sets your personal shields in place to protect you from outside energies hindering your pathway.

As for the shadow self, it's like anti-matter compared with the rest of you, and if it attempts to interact, it can be extremely chaotic and poisonous. Your etheric shield must always protect you from your shadow awakening since it is your past, you of one nanosecond ago and back through time.

GM: Any of the following symptoms indicate that your shadow self has already awakened: you feel a welling of darkness from within that can't be removed with the cleansing tools shared in this book; parts of yourself are vicious and want to take over, even though you know it's not the true you; you have a feeling of being shadowed when there's no one in flesh or spirit behind you.

AT': If your shadow self has awakened, ask the choir of angels to sing it back to sleep, and make sure all tears or weak spots in your etheric shields are repaired so it can no longer notice the present you.

The more in tune you become with your whole self, the greater your reach and depths of experiences on your journey. The reason I left this exercise for the end of the book is because you must know yourself before being able to do this easily. To remove the divisions, call on your Core Self, as well as Neraphasea and the Holy Spirit, to help identify the barriers and follow the steps below.

1. When the barriers have been identified, ask the pure light quicksilver to ignite in and around them, shattering them and vacuuming them up from the inside out and outside in.
2. Once the removal has begun, it's important that the Holy Spirit remove all ALPs that have been clinging to them, and that the Neraphasea help you reclaim any inners or suppressed parts of self.
3. After this has begun, ask Archangel Michael to ensure that anything not truly you is removed, helping him by rebirthing your personal shields.

Exploring Beyond the Material

AT': This exercise goes beyond the regions of our universe, taking you beyond the "I am all that is" being whom many people believe to be God. I say this so you understand that the "I Am" is limited to here, since it is the united mind of all life within this universe, whereas the True Creator is everywhere out beyond and loves other places as much as He/She loves here.

Once you have reclaimed your inner core and cleared some of the things hindering growth, you may wish to explore the places where your particles help anchor you within existence. These particles can be found in other realms and realities of existence, each with a life of its own. You may have unconsciously tapped into these other lives during dreams when you or they had knowledge that needed sharing. Some may live nearly identically to you, but with slight variations that set them apart. Others live very differently from you and can be of the opposite gender, a different age, and even have non-human shapes. Although the lives of these other particles don't directly influence you or each other, they have influence through unconscious thoughts and can appear as dreams or desires. That being said, when you consciously focus outward and through their eyes, you can directly influence their actions and reactions to their worlds, so be careful when doing this. It's better to focus on them from a place outside their bodies, viewing them and their worlds as spirit, rather than entering their flesh. From an external vantage point, you can still explore your greater whole and understand these particle selves, without directly influencing them until you understand their world and lives.

The following exercise can be modified for either use, but is written to prevent you from entering into their flesh.

1. Relax and breathe deeply as you climb to the top of your high space.
2. When you reach the top, call those guides and Guardian Angels whom you trust to keep you safe, and tell them that you intend to stretch yourself beyond this material realm.
3. Repeat this phrase three times: "I seek a thread to follow outward to one of my particle selves, where I can learn new things about

myself, or help those parts of me which anchor me within existence. Once I am there, that thread will stop before I enter into that particle self's personal space. I know that the thread is part of me and will always lead me home."

4. Now follow that thread. See it shine in your mind's eye and know that it will always lead you truly. Know that you are protected and that no outsider can hinder your journey, but your inner core may if it deems you unready. If your inner core tries to stop you, ask if it is appropriate for it to do so. If it answers that it *is* appropriate for you to attempt this journey now, call on the Holy Spirit to take these hesitant parts of yourself, calve them away as ALPs to allow you freedom to grow.

5. If you follow the thread and reach the world of one of your particle selves, spend time watching and understanding before attempting to interact and influence that part of you.

6. Once you have explored to your heart's content and are ready to come home, simply open your eyes and rebalance within your flesh. Have no fear of being stuck out beyond, even if you've been exploring through the eyes of your particle selves, since here is where you are anchored in flesh. Enjoy.

Appendices

The purpose of these lists is to go into detail about things which would
be too confusing in the main text. There's no need to memorize these
lists, but read through them so your subconscious mind knows them and
your Guardian Angels understand what you mean when you give
permission for cleansings.

Appendix 1:
Wrongful Uses of Power

AT': These things are created by thought focus and/or emotion, with or without the need for trinkets or other magical props. All the following must be named, rejected, and removed completely. Whether you believe in such things or not, note that you may have been bound by them in past lives when you perhaps did believe in them. Also, since they can bind your genetic line if one of your ancestors was bound, they could have warped you since conception. Call on Archangel Michael, the Holy Spirit, and all appropriate to act when dealing with their removal from yourself, and all other family members, past, present, and future who might be affected by them.

1. Spell: Binding wrongfully created with a piece of the creator of the spell's awareness (ALP) within it to tend to it. Note that these can follow souls through many lifetimes until rejected and removed.
2. Hex: Woven binding of protection, also with ALPs tending to it.
3. Curse: Binding interwoven with spells or focused thought, wrongfully choking off a person's silver cord.
4. Amulet: Object bound by a spell (with ALP) that may gain awareness of its own.
5. Emerald Verse: Chant which weaves bindings around a place to focus natural powers. This wrongfully blocks the earth's natural control.
6. Jesu Charm: Items of religious significance empowered by ALPs of their worshippers.
7. Talisman: Consciously created with focus, but no ALPs, to guide people in a certain direction.
8. Moon Madness: What happens when an unprotected person touches a power object, powered by spells so ancient they have calved away from the original spell.
9. Flesh-Bound Spell: Bio-machines clinging to people, using ALPs to hinder others.

10. Resonance Spell: Bindings using focus instead of ALPs, tuned to certain brainwaves, which trigger the spell's creator to focus on the person bound.

11. Web of Command: Webs of power bound in place by ALPs to force power to flow in a certain direction.

12. Slave Circuits: ALPs trapped in a Web of Command like living computers to focus other people's psi powers.

13. Watchers of the Dawn: Pure ALPs who have been bound by alien spells to feed the human resonance of Slave Circuits.

14. Wards: Blocks holding ALPs set in place to prevent all but the *worthy* from proceeding.

15. Evil Eye: Binding shaped with focus to cause harm or bad luck to the recipient.

+1. Those Who Tend the Above: Wrongfully focused beings of all generations who have rejected the truth of themselves in favor of wrongful actions.

Appendix 2:
Types of Beings in Existence

AT': Note that all who are mentioned here must be cleaned, healed, and returned to their appropriate places to do their true jobs, fulfilling the reason they were created by God.

1. Pure Awareness: Without shape or form, these beings have gravity due to their DNA, and true jobs list they were born with from the Creator. Their place of residence is beyond the reality realms.

2. Pure Spirit: Awareness with spirit, conscious, and ego layers anchoring them in the reality realms. Examples: angels, demons, regionals, legions, archangels, etc. If found within the reality realm or between realms, shields between realities must be called on to push these beings back to their appropriate places.

3. Human Soul: Awareness with all fifteen layers. Not all human souls have human shapes, but all have human minds. Examples: humans, aliens, trees, raptors, and toothed whales. Found nearly everywhere in existence. If these are not in flesh, but clinging or overlapping someone in flesh, or if they are found wandering without flesh, call on Archangel Michael to clean and heal them, and guide them into the Light.

4. Sibling Soul: Awareness with all fifteen layers, but accessing only ego, spirit, conscious, etheric, and material in this reality realm. Elsewhere, they have dominant realms where they can access all their layers. Examples: stars, planets, animals, plants, insects, fish, etc. When not in flesh, deal with them similarly to a human soul, above.

5. Quark: Awareness with all fifteen layers, but focused in and between the atomic and three largest micro-micron layers. Examples: Most symbionts, bacteria, viruses, mosses, etc. Archangel Raphael is the one to call on to deal with these.

6. Creature: Awareness with all fifteen layers, bound to all realities, but focused in one at a time through shifting perspective.

Examples: Elementals, mythical creatures, etc. Most of these can be dealt with by calling on appropriate guides and teachers to go to them. If this doesn't work, call on Archangel Michael. If they are young ones of their kind, you can also call on their parents and ask that the parents deal with them appropriately. Once they're gone, establish an energy barrier to prevent them from returning.

7. Micrococcus ('Coccus): Awareness with all fifteen layers, scavenger-predators that act in and between layers, realms, etc. to clean and cull. Examples: mold, fungus, rodents, coyotes, some symbionts, etc. Raphael also deals with these.

8. Micro-Micron (Micro'): Awareness with all fifteen layers, warrior/protectors that act in and between layers, realms, etc. to keep the 'coccus in check. Examples: cats, white blood cells, lions, wolves, most symbionts, etc. Also for Raphael or Michael to deal with.

9. Mitochondria (Mito'): Awareness with all fifteen layers, found within all the layers of all spirits and souls and possessing a united mind. They are connected to each other even in death, and survive the death of their host for approximately two weeks. Here too, Raphael is the one to call on.

10. Shadow: These are not the soul's shadow layer, but are born to shadow all layers of a soul to cause trouble. These are second-generation souls, and all their layers must be found and united before they can be taken by the Holy Spirit.

11. Doppelganger: Also second-generation souls created in sets of fifteen-plus-one to haunt and hinder each human soul born on Earth during the Angel Wars. Examples: doubles, puppet selves, sometimes perceived as gremlins, etc. Once found, their complete sets must be gathered in, but not united before the Holy Spirit deals with them, for they are individuals, siblings.

12. Phantom: Again, second-generation souls created to hinder us, with complete sets of layers which must be found and united so the Holy Spirit can deal with them. Of the second-generation souls, these are one of the few who have a purpose here, and have legions of their own within the light.

13. Baks: Awareness with all fifteen layers, these are true shape-changers, the first-born in a universe, with the job of shaping stars and planets, and preparing for the life forms which are to come. Examples: watchers, sentinels, and some dragons. Call on Archangel Michael to deal with those who cause trouble.

14. Parasite: Awareness with all fifteen layers who drain energy from their hosts to propagate, but seldom kill their hosts. Found attached in or between all layers of the host. See Chapter 2 for instructions on their removal.

15. Alternate: A second-generation awareness with all layers, created in wrongful timelines or loops to recreate everyone in the original timeline. These must be given over to the Holy Spirit.

+1. Fragment: These are second-generation ALPs born consciously or during stress or trauma from the parent awareness. A natural process, they are part of God's way of ensuring there will always be future generations to fill existence. When they cling to the parent awareness, they cause trouble and must be handed over to the Holy Spirit.

Appendix 3:
The Base Layers of Our Bodies

AT': All base layers have inner layers in the same number and with the same names as the base layers, just inwardly turned. A good example is to equate the base layers with things like the heart, skin, nerves, etc., with the inner layers as the cells which build the heart, skin, nerves, etc. This is just an example, since the material layer is the base layer for the heart, skin, nerves, etc., including our cells. Base layers are anchors that allow us to exist within existence, since existence consists of refined and condensed energies.

The base layers are listed here from the lightest particle to the heaviest, noting they are all of equal importance, even though the material layer is the only temporary part of us.

+1. Awareness: This is the "I source" giving you your sense of identity and awareness of your place in existence. Essence of gravity. Pewter helps focus energies of the I, and gravity helps you know yourself. *This is the layer we were born with from the Creator's own awareness.*

1. Spirit: This is the "truth source" giving you awareness and the ability to coordinate all your layers. Essence of passion. Gold helps focus the energies of truth and passion to achieve your goals.

2. Conscious: This is the "place source" giving you self-perceptions and time's perspective. Essence of focus. Silver helps focus the energies of place and focus within the vastness of time.

3. Ego: This is the "courage source" giving you ties to your place in existence. Essence of solidity. Salt helps focus energies of courage and solidity, so you know where you are within the reality realms.

The above layers are owned by all spirits, who gain the layers below only if they choose to become flesh bound.

4. Void: This is the "material source" giving your subconscious help in creating what your mind conceives. Essence of chaos. Smoky quartz helps focus energies of material and chaos to manifest your surroundings and that which you desire.

5. Memory: This is the "forms source" giving you a record of your karmic wheel and both your genetic and soul roots. Essence of common sense. Topaz helps focus the energies of form and common sense in balancing your DNA and soul tendencies.

6. Dream: This is the "creative source" giving you messages, lessons, and problem-solving techniques. Essence of chance. Red-gold zircon helps focus the energies of creativity and chance to help you sort and deal with what comes your way.

7. Thought: This is the "intuitive source" giving you messages from self and/or outsiders. Essence of patterns. Jasper helps focus the energies of intuition and patterns to help you wield free will choice in dealing with inner desires or urgings from others.

8. Emotion: This is the "empathic source" giving you warnings, directions, and motivations. Essence of conscience. Green chalcedony helps focus the energies of empathy and conscience to guide you safely through the maze of life.

9. Soul: This is the "love source" animating all your layers. Essence of flavor. Sapphire helps focus the energies of love and flavor to draw you forward along your true pathway.

10. Mind: This is the "choice source" giving you the ability to focus all layers for one goal. Essence of sequence. Emerald helps focus the energies of choice and sequence so that you can see the aftermath of your choices and how they relate to your goals.

11. Subconscious: This is the "judgment source" helping create what the mind conceives. Essence of will. White beryl helps focus the energies of judgment and will to give you the strength and determination to achieve your goals.

12. Shadow: This is the "conscience source" shaped by all bodies of your past, including who you were a nanosecond ago. Essence of set. Obsidian helps focus the energies of conscience and set to anchor you to your past lessons so you can continue forward.

13. Etheric: This is the "mine source" giving you energy and protecting your body and space perspective. Essence of shield. Agate helps focus the energies of mine and shield to protect you from your shadow layers as you continue forward along your true pathway.

14. Astral: This is the "guard source" giving you energy and protecting your soul and perspective. Essence of shield. Clear quartz helps focus the energies of guard and shield to help you know yourself apart from others.

15. Material: This is the "focus source" giving your present body focus in the direction perspective. Essence of desire. Amethyst helps focus the energies of focus and desire so you can choose which direction you wish to observe or follow.

Appendix 4:
Paradox Directional Selves (PDSs)

AT': PDSs are similar to ALPs, but are both male and female, and appropriate within the self until your future self manifests within present self to ignite you within the True Creator's First Dream. When working appropriately, they help us stay balanced and following our true pathways. When unbalanced, they cause a variety of problems and must be dealt with firmly, but with gentleness and compassion. If they are unbalanced, wrap them in the pure light quicksilver, call on the Holy Spirit and the ivy of Saint Peter's gate to help gather them in. Next, create a box from the pure light quicksilver and line it with thick velvet to protect them from harm. Place the PDS in the box and set it just outside your inner core where outsiders can't harm it. The PDS will still be able to whisper thoughts to you that are appropriate, but inappropriate thoughts will not be able to escape the box.

Here is a list of PDSs, where they are found, and what they do when balanced and unbalanced:

1. Chancellor of Self: This is found *within* the particles of self and is born to focus you on research, inside and out, needed to expand current knowledge. Out of balance it creates distractions that hinder your ability to focus on what is needed for growth.

2. Vizier of Self: This is found *beneath* the particles of self and is born to watch over teachers and teachings, checking what they pass on against your inner knowing. Out of balance it allows falsehoods to be taught without checking for the truth.

3. Seneschal of Self: This is found *beside* the particles of self and is born to be the gatekeeper of knowledge and growth, sorting truth from deception within new knowledge and what others teach. Out of balance it refuses access to knowing and knowledge that would allow inner growth.

4. Chamberlain of Self: This is found *behind* the particles of self and is born to regulate clear sight to see self and those around you.

Out of balance it distorts the view and can even refuse to see self and others clearly, favoring fantasies and deceptions.

5. Viceroy of Self: This is found *before* the particles of self and is born to challenge new codes of conduct to ensure they work with your true pathway. Out of balance it rejects new codes of conduct, regardless of whether they are appropriate.

6. Chancellor-Regent of Self: This is found *between* the particles of self and is born to balance the hopes and desires of the future self. Out of balance it creates doubt, indecision, and causes instability that may manifest as mental illness.

7. Vizier-Regent of Self: This is found *left* of the particles of self and is born to hold you to the highest standard of your future self. Out of balance it sabotages attempts to achieve and maintain those high standards.

8. Seneschal-Regent of Self: This is found *above* particles of self and is born to regulate curiosity and fascination with new subjects. Out of balance it punishes curiosity with fear of the unknown or different.

9. Chamberlain-Regent of Self: This is found *around* the particles of self and is born to help unravel mysteries and puzzles, including past life carry-overs. Out of balance it accentuates these and creates puzzles from things that should be easily understood.

10. Viceroy-Regent of Self: This is found *outside* the particles of self and is born to command self-control and self-respect, ensuring they allow lessons to be learned. Out of balance they short circuit these and uphold habits and addictions beyond the lessons learned.

11. Chancellor-Arbiter of Self: This is found in the *here* particles of self and is born to challenge perceptions of self as you are pressed forward into future self. Out of balance it distorts perceptions of self so you believe you are what others believe you to be.

12. Vizier-Arbiter of Self: This is found in *future* particles of self and is born to challenge the inner core's view of reality. Out of balance it raises questions that confuse perceptions of reality, hindering true sight and clear thinking.

13. Seneschal-Arbiter of Self: This is found in the *now* particles of self and is born to regulate compassion for self and others, allowing empathy to guide, but not control, choices. Out of balance it creates chaos by intensifying emotions and hindering clear sight.

14. Chamberlain-Arbiter of Self: This is found *right* of particles of self and is born to stimulate courage without thought when needed. Out of balance it causes unreasonable fear or causes one to act where no action is needed.

15. Viceroy-Arbiter of Self: This is found in *past* particles of self and is born to renew faith in your perceptions of self and why you are here. Out of balance it causes you to believe you have no right to be here and may cause suicidal tendencies.

+1. Regent-Arbiter of Self: This is found in *center* particles of self and is born to challenge life lessons when lessons have already been learned. Out of balance it forgets lessons already learned causing you to repeat them endlessly.

Appendix 5:
Objects and Energy Forms

AT': Once found and rejected, these things must be cleaned away by Archangel Michael and the Holy Spirit, then dissolved and vacuumed up, from the inside out and outside in, into the pure light where they will be recycled.

1. Scaffolding: Created from old essence, in and between layers, it hinders growth and allows hiding places for ALPs and outsiders.
2. False Time: See Appendix 9 for complete list.
3. Essence: Psychic sweat of self and/or others, this is natural and can deliver messages from one layer of the self to another. However, it causes problems when it lingers after its job is done.
4. Wrongful Powers: See Appendix 1 for complete list.
5. Objects: Shaped from old essence or other crud by outsiders, these can be found in or between layers, as well as outside the self. Created by those wishing to hide in or beneath them, objects can take the form of eggs, statues, buildings, etc.
6. Karmic Crud: Even when karmic ties have been forgiven and released, crud can remain behind the tie.
7. Atrophied Pieces of Self: These are parts of self that have died due to prolonged overlapping by outsiders and/or ALPs.
8. Illusions: Projections of self or others which hinder true sight due to focus, preconceptions, deceptions, etc. These must be recognized before they can be rejected and cleared away.
9. Vibration: From outside the self, these can interfere with the self's own vibration and cause both mental and physical illness.
10. Creations: Similar to objects, but more complex, these machines, weapons, etc., can transmute energies for the purpose of hindering others.
11. Trash: Slime, sludge, crud, etc., shaped from stray particles of old essence when outsiders overlap a person.

12. Energy Forms: Energy shaped into various objects to hinder the self and/or others in existence.

13. Energy Beings: Created to mock or duplicate a being, either to protect self or hinder others. These must be vacuumed into the pure light as soon as their appropriate tasks are complete, otherwise they hinder self and others.

14. Bio-Machines: Created by off-worlders to hide in or influence a being, these can only be dealt with by binding them in pure light and blocking their energy flow, i.e., by killing off the biological elements in them. Only then can they be vacuumed and cleansed away.

15. Blocks: Walls, barriers, veils, blinders, etc., which prevent growth. These can be caused by the self, the subconscious, or outsiders, and can follow us through and between lifetimes.

+1. Traps: Set in situations of society, marriage, karmic crossroads, tests of growth, etc., these can be triggered by your choices, or can blind you to all but one choice due to your mindset.

Appendix 6:
Wrongful Attachments

AT': To deal with any of these, call on Archangel Michael and all appropriate Wild Cards to act in all ways appropriately.

1. Layering: This is when beings layer into another being's particles to hide, influence, or confuse them.

2. Clinging: This is when beings cling to the outside of another being's particles to hide, influence, or confuse them.

3. Bindings: This is when beings block another being's connections to their power webs to influence or confuse them.

4. Spells: This is when beings block the connections between another being's power objects and webs to influence or confuse them.

5. Nets: This is when beings block the energy flow between the Creator's organs and a being's power objects, preventing the energy from reaching them and allowing for influence or confusion.

6. Strands: Beings attach these to other beings' silver cords as they pass between the realms, building greater bodies to influence or confuse them.

7. Webs: Beings attach these to other beings' silver cords as they pass between the layers, building greater bodies to influence or confuse them.

8. Poison: Beings use their negative micro-micron essence particles between the inner layers of other beings to influence or confuse them.

9. Knot: Beings use their mental strands to tie off parts of other beings' power webs, blocking the flow to influence or confuse them.

10. Pick: These are like ice picks, formed from the conscious demands of beings shoved into other being's web modifiers to influence or confuse them.

11. Nuzzle: When beings snuggle against other beings's power objects to influence or confuse them.

12. Lynch: When beings use other beings' thought patterns to try to strangle them into being influenced or confused.

13. Sex: When beings use their sexual chakras to stimulate other beings' memory pods into action to influence or confuse them.

14. Jumble: Confusion created when beings use their will power to block other beings' web modifiers from processing the energies passing through them to influence or confuse them.

15. Corral: When beings fence other beings from their power web connections to influence or confuse them.

+1. Pocket: When beings cling to other beings using scars or karmic ties like a pocket to cling close, camouflaged, to hide, influence, or confuse.

Appendix 7:
Blocks to the Truth

AT': By blocks to the truth, I mean both those that come from outside, and those that your own mind locks into due to your worldview, or the simple refusal to grow beyond your comfort zone.

1. False Assumptions: Taking part of an incident or fact, and building false information around it, without realizing it is wrong.

2. Self-Deceptions: Knowing the truth of an incident or event, and building false information around it to ignore the truth.

3. Wrongful Knowledge: False assumptions created by others that are passed on and accepted as true knowledge.

4. Nutation Hither: Involuntary scattering of attention and focus, perhaps caused by the subconscious refusal to allow the conscious mind to see.

5. Irritating Pride: When pride, either justified or not, is used wrongfully, blocking growth and knowledge, or hindering the growth of someone else.

6. Just Pity: Pity, whether justified or not, always harms the receiver as well as the giver. It's better to understand what is needed and give help, or walk away knowing help is not wanted.

7. Deserving Laughter: Laughter to relieve stress is only good when the stressed being is the one who initiates the laughter.

8. Dumb Enjoyment: Something done for physical pleasure or momentary gratification, while knowing it to be wrong. This includes all types of enjoyment that cause harm to self or others.

9. Blind Fight: Reacting with aggression without knowledge of the situation, or ignoring the truths to push a falsehood.

10. Unwarranted Dignity: Acting more dignified than your layers or soul want you to act.

11. False Fossae: Pitfalls that trap you in ruts and block sight of the truth.

12. Closed Ears: Complete rejection of anything new or which disagrees with what you were taught to believe is truth.

13. Hard Multiplicity: Having a hard time doing many things at once due to blockage.
14. Jib Histaminase: Balking at clearing away invaders to the system.
15. Clenched Fist: Unwillingness to accept truths that are offered.
+1. Indifferent Mitos: When the mitochondria no longer care about the layers they help support.

Appendix 8:
Emotional Roots to Physical Pain, Disease, or Illness

GM & AT': Below are examples provided to us by Archangels Raphael and Michael denoting the effect our emotions can have on our physical being. Focus on the situation(s) occurring when the pain started, and use the commands in the book to release the emotions.

Physical Pain	Emotional Possibilities	Other Possibilities
- neck pain	- who is a pain in your neck? - fear of your past? of growth?	- lost spirits clinging to you - someone focusing negative intent on you - mitochondria out of balance or concerned
- general back pain	- frustration at being unable to maneuver through life - fear of failure at the tasks you've chosen	- need to stand tall and claim your truths - need for you to hold your head up and strive to be who you were born to be
- lower back pain	- money is a constant concern - anger at being stuck in a job situation	- birthing new desires or possibilities - taking on more then you're willing to carry
- middle back pain	- guilt over situation(s) in your life - frustration at not being able to help more	- being pushed into situations not appropriate for you - compassion preventing you from saying something to others which needs to be said
- upper back pain	- stress, weight of the world on your shoulders - anger at the injustices around you	- inability to prioritize - too focused on a single subject rather than seeing the whole

- heartburn, nausea	- anger or fear at self, something, or someone - frustration needing direction into action	- your body trying to stop you from doing something not appropriate - part of the fight or flight response
- headache	- denial of self or others for who you/they are	- opening or overload of spiritual connections - negative psychic energy nearby
- ears	- anxiety triggered by vibrations around you - fear of something you don't want to hear or listen to	- angelic singing too loud or vibrant - cleansing of ears so you can hear spirit (right) or Elementals (left)
- throat	- angry or fearful words not said - doubts or low self worth cause you to swallow what you want to say	- lymphatic symbionts warning of body out of balance or impending illness - throat chakra clogged and hindering health
- teeth	- discomfort with decisions needing to be made or that you have made - fear of memories that are surfacing to be dealt with	- rebalancing of past, present, and future - challenges to self worth because of karmic bindings

Any pain can signify something wrong, i.e., psychic parasites, something clinging or overlapping your personal space, karmic energy surfacing from an old wound, pseudo-Wild Cards surfacing that need to be claimed, which means the area around them needs to be cleansed. The side you feel the pain on could also be a clue that it's something you're refusing acceptance of (left side if right handed, opposite if left handed), something you need for growth or releasing (right side if right handed, opposite if left), or something that's hindering growth. In previous chapters, you'll find the various cleansing commands to deal with these.

Remember that your emotions can create negative energy in your body, that in turn creates physical weakness. You might say you hurt your knee by turning it the wrong way, or that it's hereditary, but the illness or pain wouldn't happen unless you already have weakness there.

Also remember that before negative energy can manifest as serious pain, disease, or illness, there has to be a lot of it, which means one release may not rid you of all pain, but continuous releases of the negative energy should help.

Medical doctors and psychiatrists or psychologists have their work to do too, so don't hesitate to ask for their help when necessary.

Appendix 9:
False Time

AT': All false time is wrong, effectively confusing and distorting true time. If you find false time, call on the Holy Spirit and Archangel Michael to surround it with pure light, cleanse whatever awarenesses are within it, and vacuum the false time from the outside in and the inside out into the pure light for recycling.

1. Fragments: Fragmented time is created when an ALP is calved away from the parent awareness by trauma. Time continues to move forward, but along a very narrow pathway which splinters every time the ALP steps away from their parent's true pathway into the True Creator's First Dream.

2. Loops: Time loops occur when a being experiences a trauma so great that the ALP it calves rejects the forward motion of time, continually jerking backwards to the beginning of the situation which led to the trauma. They repeat the event, not remembering, and always wanting a different ending.

3. Alternatives: Alternate time occurs when time travels forward at a normal pace, but space has altered, splintering away from the original because the ALP rejects an action dealing with a great number of beings.

4. Creations: Created time occurs when a being seeks to create a conduit reaching beyond their own regions of existence, rendering them blind to true time as they focus their energies elsewhere, birthing an ALP and recreating all the life they sense in this other space.

5. Illusions: Time illusions occur when a being feels the need for more or less time in which to move. Focused unconsciously on the desire to slow or speed time, this can create a pocket of false time that travels with the being, populated by an ALP whom the parent awareness focuses through. Although it keeps pace with true time, those within the bubble experience time at a slower or faster pace.

6.   Passes: Time passes are passageways through time that don't touch time; these are consciously created by those who seek easier paths from one place to another, but only ALPs travel them, not the parent awareness. They travel through false time into false space.

7.   Voids: Time voids are places where there is no time or pathway, created by a being's rejection of true time, which creates an ALP who stagnates.

8.   Twists: Time twists turn time back around and behind itself to interfere with true time, but it is only the ALP and alternates (created duplicates of everyone in the region) within it who suffer.

9.   Warps: Time warps are used by some beings to try to jump forward along the time stream, passing over vast stretches and coming out into a false future, created by their own unconscious desires. Alternates are created to fill the roles of those the being believes it will find, while the ALP of that being retains the main focus of the being. The body still exists in true time, sometimes in a coma.

10. Kinks: Time kinks are blockages in the normal flow of time. These happen when a being tries to hide, consciously wrapping time around themselves and refusing to flow with it. Note that this does not involve ALPs or alternates. The being must be gathered in, healed, and taught that its reasons for hiding are no longer there.

11. Pockets: Time pockets occur when a spirit leaves its appropriate region and enters another where time doesn't flow in the same manner. The spirit must be found and returned to its appropriate region.

12. Events: Time events are cruxes in the path. When they occur naturally, they serve the First Dream Pathways, but when they are created by beings, they can distort the truth of the future, leading beings down false paths.

13. Spells: Time spells are created by those who wish to bind others to their will, distorting other being's perceptions of time to control their movements. This creates a bubble of false time that travels with the being, but keeps pace with true time. Those in the bubble experience time differently from those outside it.

14. Stains: Time stains don't stop the normal flow of time, but unconsciously bind a being to the emotions surrounding a traumatic event, triggered by memory. The memory must be recognized and healed so the stain can be cleansed.

15. Smudges: Time smudges are similar to stains, except they bind a being to the essence of a traumatic event even after healing has occurred. Karmic ties are involved and must be forgiven before healing and cleansing can be completed.

+1. Paradox: Paradox time, when used by the True Creator, helps us achieve our place in the First Dream, but when used by deceivers, or those who wish to hinder others, it can trigger any of the other types of false time. Paradox time occurs when something in the future manifests in the past, altering the time line. True time doesn't change, but time splinters off in other directions creating ALPs and alternates. The *only* paradox time that didn't do this was the First Dream which, when sent backwards into time, went outside and before time existed. That is what awoke the True Creator and set Him/Her to creating existence and all those seen within the Dream. *We are all ALPs of the True Creator existing within the paradox of time created by our future selves.*

Appendix 10:
Inner Core Parts of the Self

AT': What follows is a list of parts of the self and the inner core objects and organs that refine the raw powers of existence for our use. Everything listed below sprouts from the Core Self to give you shape and substance in existence.

1.   Inner Self: Inner core objects and the karma organ, both shaped like tunnels, feed us subconscious energy.

2.   Seeker Self: Inner "I" object and the possibility organ, both shaped like flat diamonds, feed us thought energy.

3.   Higher Self: Inner awareness object and the aware organ, both shaped like round nets, feed us conscious energy. This is our ancestral mind.

4.   Inner Child: Inner voice object and the focus organ, both shaped like spider webs, feed us ego energy. Note that this is not the same as the inners spoken of in Chapter 5 that are in need of reclaiming.

5.   Hidden Self: Inner space object and the shield organ, both shaped like clusters of light, feed us astral energy.

6.   Command Self: Inner feeling object and the base organ, both shaped like spirals, feed us emotion energy.

7.   Blind Self: Inner essence object and the echo organ, both shaped like mirrors without edges, reflecting anything approaching them, feed us soul energy.

8.   My Self: Inner body object and the shield organ, both shaped like buttons and corresponding to the fifteen-plus chakras threaded together by the kundalini, feed us etheric energy.

9.   I Am Self: Inner craving object and the stray organ, both shaped like the eternity symbol reaching across the horizon, feed us material energy. This is also the self that anchors within the "I Am Being" who unites all minds in this universe and whom some people mistakenly believe to be God.

10. True Pathway Self: Inner choice object and the power organ,

both shaped like trees, feed us memory energy.

11. Remembered Self: Inner shadow and the unconscious organ, both shaped like pools of water with changing shorelines, feed us shadow energy. Note that this is the only safe way to interact with our shadow self, since the shadow isn't aware of us as we do this.

12. New Self: Inner dream object and the fluctuation organ, both shaped like boxes, feed us dream energy.

13. Highest Self: Inner self object and the manage organ, both shaped like sheets of light, feed us spirit energy.

14. Challenged Self: Inner warrior object and the roots organ, both shaped like flowers, feed us void energy.

15. Only Self: Inner command object and the command organ, both shaped like spheres, feed us mind energy.

+1. True Self: Inner tree object and the blood organ, both shaped like tree branches giving the mitos access to us, feeds us awareness energy. This is the mitos' group mind.

Appendix 11:
True Creator's First Dream

AT': *In the Beginning, there was a Dream...* In the beginning there was nothingness, empty yet full of potential. There's no telling how long this lasted since time did not yet exist. The void churned with possibilities, but not reality, expectant, waiting, as if preparing to give birth. Then a sound echoed through the vastness, opening the way for a vision to flash through the nothingness, filling it for three nanoseconds, disturbing the churning mass of nothingness, burning its image on it so deeply and clearly that God awoke.

Calling forth the vision that had awakened Him/Her, God looked down and saw a horse rearing in majestic beauty on a high plateau of lush turquoise colored grass. The black stallion's hide was speckled with clumps of swirling gold and silver galaxies, and his eyes shone with the wisdom of the ages. Seeing the creature, God loved its beauty and grace, rejoicing in its purity of spirit and named him the Cosmic Stallion.

A rainbow colored sky looked down upon the plateau, and a large cathedral-like building attracted His/Her attention. It was shaped from deep red rock which had once been wood, and was set back from the edge of the cliff on a rise so the occupants could see the sky's reflection in the ocean below, if they chose to look. Stretching back and away from the cliff, a large area was marked off by marble slabs large enough to be the resting place for twelve ships of all shapes and forms. These ships were infants compared to the giant mother ships floating nearly motionless far above the planet, yet each made the stallion appear minute.

Looking inside the building, which was a ship in and of itself, God found beings from twelve different races, with all members of each race focusing through a single member of its people standing in the building. One being stood alone, representing her race with the power of all her race burning in her eyes, the faith and love within her keeping her safe among these strangers. God could feel the group consciousness of each race focused through these twelve minds, with the glow of many more races looking on.

These souls were representative of their people, coming from the twelve directions of their galaxy. God could feel the twelve channeling trillions of souls, all calling out to Him/Her in one moment, stirring Him/Her out of silence and into awareness of Self. Their voices sang out different notes, carrying across time and distance to Him/Her, awakening Him/Her with His/Her true name. Although each of the twelve voices called out a different name, they were all His/Hers, all true, all causing the void to echo their truth. There were also three voices from beyond those twelve that could be seen, three voices which came from within, between, and around these others, so minute He/She had to focus deep within the vision to see them. They prayed that He/She would guide them in uniting the cosmos and bringing peace to its diverse people. They begged Him/Her to show them the way into the future and prosperity as they named Him/Her, demanding that He/She come to them. Then they called out a question that was cut short as the third nanosecond ended, and God was left alone once more but for this vision.

Pondering the vision, God realized they were beings from the twelve directions of a cosmos that did not yet exist. Galaxies filled with life that had not yet come into being. Life so rich and powerful they had created a paradox of time, which called time itself into being as God awoke. There was something else that occurred during the three nanoseconds of that vision that God began to think of as a dream, the First Dream. As God was vibrating with the energy flowing through that paradox of time, He/She could almost see what had occurred before, almost saw before He/She had existed. God ached to recapture those nanoseconds and discover if He/She was truly the first being to exist, or if in fact there was someone even more ancient who had created Him/Her.

Glimpsing purpose in the void, purpose in the vision beyond that which these twelve plus three races wished for, God decided to create the dream and the beings in it. He/She would guide them to that rainbow planet where they would call out to Him/Her, uniting the powers of their cosmos and triggering the paradox of time. Hungering for the richness of it, God focused His/Her desires and emotions on bringing them to the moment when they had this power to awaken time itself, so He/She could reach back before then, and see if He/She was the first being or if others existed before. With the vision no more than an image recorded in His/Her being, God realized that He/She was alone and lonely. He/She could see nothing beyond Him/Herself, nor within, except for that vision from the future. God knew then that the only way He/She could see beyond His/Her own existence was to make that vision a reality. For only those beings, born of God, part of Him/Her, could call forth the power God needed to see the truth of before. When they came together, they would hold the power to help God look beyond Him/Herself to see God's own creator, and discover if there were more like Him/Herself.

From that vision, the First Dream, one thing burned clearly in God's mind. One race rose above all others in power and potential, in beauty and in darkness. This race, smaller than most, weaker than all, would either lead the other races in their quest for the truth, or destroy them. Disturbed by the darkness of this race, God also knew they were the only hope for seeing beyond Him/Herself, for there was something that set them apart from the others. It was the human hearts' and minds' grasp of the powers of paradox that had awakened Him/Her within the void, leading the others backwards through time to that first nanosecond. The human soul had led the way, even as one had led the gathering.

Well, now you know what triggered God to create us and existence. He/She wanted to recreate that vision, that First Dream. So the foundations of existence were shaped from refined power and God calved or birthed awareness from His/Her own being to populate the realities, realms, and that which lies between. Of course, things didn't work out perfectly at first and time imploded fifteen times before coming to this point here and now, but that too was part of destiny since it added texture and flavor to existence. Before we were given life in the flesh, life was rich and full out beyond, in the spirit realms where the angels reside. When speaking of the big bang, the first nanoseconds of existence in this universe, only the material layers are spoken of. Adding all the other layers of existence to them, I found that the spirits and angels call this place the Megaverse. There are many Megaverses in the material realm, beginning as eggs that hatch into beings so vast they encompass the entire universe and are driven by a united mind, all life in the Megaverse united as one. Not wishing to complicate things, but wishing to speak the truth, I must also tell you that the united mind is growing within three universal bodies that will eventually draw apart as their time of hatching approaches. When this occurs, those of us who live in the universe will barely, if at all, notice a difference, since even separated and hatched, the united mind interweaves between the three. To see a picture of the Megaversal nest, visit my website, aunt-t-pathfinder.20m.com, and click on "A Few Eggs."

The First Dream is what the Creator desires, the reason we came into being, but it's not the "be all and end all" and isn't even necessary. The Creator doesn't need to see before His/Her own existence; He/She would like to, but can survive without doing so. What is important is the True United Destiny born from that Dream, what happens after the asking and answering of the question that ignited the paradox of time, since the True United Destiny has already been bought and paid for by antiquity's martyr, by the weight of blood she has given in martyrdom since time began. Her blood was ignited by Archangel Michael's sword of pure light and became quicksilver, melding to the Creator's pure light, and was used to pay the debts of existence, past, present, and future. Because of this, the True United Destiny is ensured, even if the question that awoke the Creator before time began is never asked or answered.

What awaits us in the future, some century in the future, is that when the loom holding the tapestry of time is full, new looms will be born to weave new tapestries. Each awareness born from the Creator, all the first-generation children, will be born outward in their own destiny eggs where they will find their ALPs awaiting them, awake and self-aware, filling all realms and realities even as we do here. Those of us who are evolved enough to be aware of this transition will find ourselves in a God-like position, able to consciously interact with them even as our Creator does with us here, but perhaps it's best if you think of yourself as the parent, not a god. Those who are less evolved will find themselves shifted into eggs with their present surroundings duplicated exactly, except those they share their surroundings with will be their own ALPs, not their siblings. They will have the chance to evolve in their own time and space. Eventually, when their own looms are full, their destiny egg will hatch. As they are born outward to be with the Creator, new looms will be born to weave the tapestries of their children, who will begin the process again, with the next generation of children born from their own awareness. After all, there are vast empty regions beyond existence that the Creator wishes to fill, and how better to do so than with countless generations of His/Her progeny?

What happens when you are born outside your destiny egg? You will be welcomed by the True Creator into a vast realm where all your desires can manifest joyfully and where you can again come together with others of your generation as you do here. Together or alone, you can create worlds to amuse yourself and explore ideas. You will be God-like, but not God, since there is always the True Creator. We will be adults, instead of the children we now are. Sound boring? Then begin thinking about what you would do. As long as it isn't harmful to yourself or others, there's no limit beyond your own ability to discover your potential.

Appendix 12:
My Basic Beliefs, by Aunt T' Pathfinder

1. I believe in a True Creator, First Being of Pre-Existence, creator of the foundations of existence, and First Parent of all life in and beyond existence who is tolerant of the religions humanity has shaped to try and understand Him/Her. I know there are many who would like to claim the title "God" who are not the True Creator, but ask them, "Who owns the longest thread on the tapestry of time?" Then ask the keepers of the tapestry of time to tell you the truth. Many regional commanders have believed they were "God" because they've never looked beyond their own regions of existence to see what else exists. Don't let them deceive you or themselves by believing other than the truth.

2. I believe that the True Creator is disappointed in us only when we use His/Her names to cause harm to others or to teach others to hate. We are all the Truth Creator's children; each of us is here for a reason, and that reason has nothing to do with hatred. The True Creator rejoices in our differences, which create the textures and flavors of life, so when you rejoice in those differences, you are worshipping the True Creator in His/Her most basic desire.

3. I believe that the True Creator birthed us from His/Her awareness to manifest the First Dream, that each of us was created to bring into being that Dream, and that within us is a template of the Dream that we strive to manifest. Each of us has a place in the First Dream no one else can fill, and no one can come into that place overlapped or controlling another, since that would hinder all involved from finding their true place.

4. I believe that everyone has the right to be alone within themselves, in command of their own true pathway, whole and healthy in mind and body, free from outside attachments that might warp clear and knowing choices, and balanced in their own inner core. Only when we are clean and free from attachments do we have clear enough sight to know our true path's choices.

5. I believe we are all unique and necessary to the True Creator to manifest pieces of the truth buried in us that join with the truths others manifest to reveal the whole truth of existence. The only way to do this is to know and trust your inner self and be able to listen to your inner knowing, trusting it to guide you truthfully even when it means doing that which your spirit guides and guardians hesitate over, since you are the only one who knows which steps you must travel to reach your true place in our True United Destiny.

6. I believe that if each of us finds those truths in ourselves and manifests them, we will activate our own unique jobs list, eliminating the need for manmade laws and judgments, that we will work together as a joyous whole to manifest our True United Destiny. This may seem an impossible task, but think about it; if we each do that which is appropriate to our pathway and allow others to follow their own pathways appropriately, how can we harm each other?

7. I believe that our mitochondria (symbionts within each cell of our bodies) have awareness and are our partners in life, second-generation children of the True Creator who have given up their independence to nurture us. We can speak with them through that part of our brain that joins our spinal column, and they are eager to help and guide us through life, companions and friends who help wherever we allow them.

8. I believe we are here to learn how to be creators so that someday we can graduate into our own realms of existence, which we will fill with our own children who will learn how to become creators even as we are doing now. In turn, these children will eventually graduate into their own realms to fill the vast expanses of void with loving joyous light and growth while we are born outward into the greater realm where we will commune with the True Creator as you now commune with your parents, as adults.

9. I believe that in the future we will join other races from across this galaxy and create a paradox of time that will reach back before time itself and awaken the True Creator from slumber and cause Him/Her to realize that He/She is alone, thus triggering the True Creator's desire to recreate the True Dream that stirred Him/Her

to awaken. Since then, the True Creator has strived to guide us into that future where the paradox of time was created.

10. I believe that each of us was granted free will as well as a hunger to manifest the First Dream, free will to find our own way into our individual places in the Dream, and the hunger to ensure it will eventually come into being. The True Creator knows the ending because of the First Dream, but not the steps each of us traveled to reach that place, which is why our free will is so important. All life has been given free will, even the spirits within the light, since they too must find their true pathway to manifest their places in the First Dream.

11. I believe that existence is vast and this universe is a tiny part of it, but an important part since it is here that the paradox of time that awoke the True Creator was born. There is life in the other realms and realities that make up existence, and we are anchored in those places to give us substance here, although here is where our focus lies since humanity is the guiding force in manifesting the paradox of time.

12. I believe that humanity is not alone in this universe or on Earth, and although some off-worlders are benign, some are dangerous, and others simply have their own agendas for humanity that hinder our true destiny. As each person must walk his or her true pathway unhindered by outsiders, so humanity must find and walk our true pathway in order to manifest the paradox of time, companions with (but not controlled by) the off-worlders among us.

13. I believe the angels and other celestial beings don't care what names we call them, or what religion we try to bind them to, since they go where they are needed to do their true jobs now that the Angel Wars are over and they are able to see their own true pathways clearly. Although the angels don't care what names we give them, they have names they prefer to be called to set them apart from others of their kind, and they will gladly tell you those names if you ask. If they refuse to give you a name, they are deceivers or self-deceivers and should be dealt with appropriately by Archangel Michael and his legions.

14. I believe our genetic ancestry is of equal importance to our soul's history, both shaping us into who we are now, but that we can only manifest our full potential by understanding both, and releasing any karmic ties or curses which might have come to us through either past. In embracing our genetic ancestry, we can access the knowledge of those ancestors through that part of our brain (right temple area). The central part of our brain gives us access to our inner knowing and to our soul's history, which we need to balance that which is passed from our ancestors.

15. I believe in the loving joyous light of growth and truth, and that each of us must demand our right to follow our true pathway and give others the freedom to follow theirs, fighting only when our own or others' pathways are infringed upon by those who wish to control us. By demanding that right and protecting it for others, we learn when it's appropriate to act, and when it's appropriate to allow others to act. The True Creator loves us unconditionally, but that doesn't mean we have the right to infringe on other beings' rights to be free and whole. This doesn't mean you should become a vegetarian or starve yourself since the souls in the plants and animals we eat have chosen that pathway for themselves to nourish us.

+1. I believe that we have strived for and failed at manifesting the paradox of time fifteen times before, only to have time implode and take us back to the beginning to try again. This has left stains and shadows on our threads in the tapestry of time caused by karma that must be dealt with as we deal with karma created during this, the final time line. Only when all karma has been acknowledged, forgiven, and cleared away will we be unbound by the past and free to move forward unhindered by those shadows.

Gail M. Blackman has a business diploma in Human Resource Management and worked in this field for over ten years. Following the birth of her second child, she chose to stay home, but continued to work in HRM teaching at a nearby college, and then online. She has spent the last five years developing, working with, and teaching people around the world the benefits of WCT. Looking back on her experiences and choices, it is very apparent that everything has led to this passion, helping others clear the way to finding their own true passion.

A private person, Aunt T' Pathfinder has reached out to the world with these teachings, so everyone has the chance to be clean inside without having to feel the pain she felt at the beginning of her own cleansing process. She has been working online to help individuals and the world become clean, but even online has noticed people falling into the trap of believing in her more than the teachings. To avoid this with others, she seeks to remain private so they will turn to the teachings and depend on themselves rather than on her. She urges you to avoid this trap by finding the strength within yourself, believing in yourself, and standing on your own two feet as you exercise free will choice.

Other Burman Books Available:

The Inner Power Series:

Intuitive Security For Women
Abundance for Life, Love and Money
For Golfers and Other Athletes
Seducing Your Man
Seducing Your Woman
Anxiety and Depression

Fiction:

Call Waiting
The Horse in the Attic

Other:

Art of Body Detoxing DVD
Healing Mind and Spirit: Introduction to Wild Card Therapy
Confessions of a Massage Parlor Princess
The Truth About Infidelity
The Ashley Madison Diaries

You are always welcome to visit
www.BurmanBooks.com